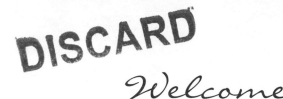

Welcome

THE
EVERYTHING®

HEALTH GUIDES

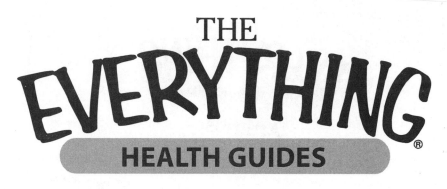

When you're faced with a pressing health issue, your first instinct is to find out as much about it as you can. With so much conflicting information out there, where can you turn for professional, supportive advice?

Packed with the most recent, up-to-date data, THE EVERYTHING® HEALTH GUIDES help ensure that you get a good diagnosis, choose the best doctor, and find the right medical treatment. With this one comprehensive resource, you and your family members have all the information you could possibly need at your fingertips.

THE EVERYTHING® HEALTH GUIDES are an extension of the bestselling Everything® series in the health category, which also includes *The Everything® Alzheimer's Book* and *The Everything® Diabetes Book*. Accessible and easy to read, THE EVERYTHING® HEALTH GUIDES provide specific details and clear examples that relate to your given medical situation. If you're looking for one-stop, all-inclusive guides that allow you to understand and become more in tune with your body, this groundbreaking series is the perfect tool for you.

Visit the entire Everything® series at *www.everything.com*

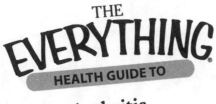

THE EVERYTHING®
HEALTH GUIDE TO
Arthritis

Dear Reader,

What a surprise—I was healthy one day and unhealthy the next. It's a day I will never forget, because no day after that was like any day that came before. I was 19 years old and coming down a flight of stairs. The pain in my legs was unlike anything I had felt before. It's amazing how quickly you can convince yourself it's nothing. My leg fell asleep in class, I first thought, or I hurt it playing tennis.

In reality, after the pain became worse instead of better, and after many diagnostic tests, my doctor told me that I had rheumatoid arthritis. That's where my journey into the world of arthritis began. I had a lot to learn, because I knew essentially nothing about arthritis and certainly didn't know any young people with arthritis.

I learned about arthritis from all the educational materials I could get my hands on. However, the best teacher of all was experience. The books can't teach you what to expect or how to live with arthritis. Though every person must decide his own best course, shared knowledge and shared experiences are powerful.

It has been more than thirty-two years since my diagnosis. My husband also has rheumatoid arthritis; we met in an arthritis support group. Arthritis has been a significant part of both of our lives and our life as a couple. Life with arthritis is not easy, but it can still be happy and fulfilling. It is my hope that this book will help you face your own challenges with the disease.

Carol Eustice http://arthritis.about.com

THE

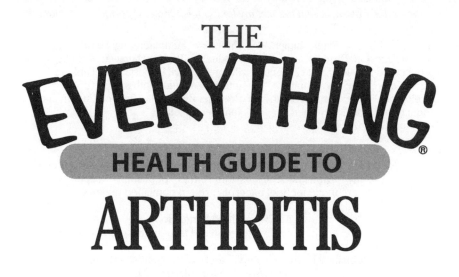

EVERYTHING®

HEALTH GUIDE TO

ARTHRITIS

Professional advice on managing
pain, choosing the right treatment,
and leading an active lifestyle

Carol Eustice
The About.com Guide to Arthritis
Technical Review by Scott J. Zashin, M.D.

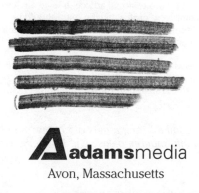

Aadamsmedia
Avon, Massachusetts

To my father, who passed away in 1986, after living bravely with scleroderma and Raynaud's disease. And to Rick, my loving husband and partner in all that I do.

• • •

Innovation Director: Paula Munier
Editorial Director: Laura M. Daly
Associate Copy Chief: Sheila Zwiebel
Acquisitions Editor: Kerry Smith
Development Editor: Katrina Schroeder
Production Editor: Casey Ebert
Technical Reviewer: Scott J. Zashin

Director of Manufacturing: Susan Beale
Production Project Manager: Michelle Roy Kelly
Prepress: Erick DaCosta, Matt LeBlanc
Interior Layout: Heather Barrett,
Brewster Brownville, Colleen Cunningham,
Jennifer Oliveira

An Everything® Series Book.
Everything® and everything.com® are registered trademarks of F+W Publications, Inc.

Published by Adams Media, an F+W Publications Company
57 Littlefield Street, Avon, MA 02322 U.S.A.
www.adamsmedia.com
ISBN 10: 1-59869-410-3
ISBN 13: 978-1-59869-410-9
Printed in the Canada.

J I H G F E D C B A

Library of Congress Cataloging-in-Publication Data
Eustice, Carol.
The everything health guide to arthritis / Carol Eustice, with Scott J. Zashin.
p. cm. – (An Everything series book)
Includes bibliographical references and index.
ISBN-13: 978-1-59869-410-9 (pbk.)
ISBN-10: 1-59869-410-3 (pbk.)
1. Arthritis–Popular works. I. Zashin, Scott J. II.
Title. RC933.E845 2007
616.7'22–dc22
2007015884

This publication is designed to provide accurate and authoritative information with regard to the subject matter covered. It is sold with the understanding that the publisher is not engaged in rendering legal, accounting, or other professional advice. If legal advice or other expert assistance is required, the services of a competent professional person should be sought.
—From a *Declaration of Principles* jointly adopted by a Committee of the American Bar Association and a Committee of Publishers and Associations

Many of the designations used by manufacturers and sellers to distinguish their products are claimed as trademarks. Where those designations appear in this book and Adams Media was aware of a trademark claim, the designations have been printed with initial capital letters.

This book is available at quantity discounts for bulk purchases.
For information, please call 1-800-289-0963.

All the examples and dialogues used in this book are fictional and have been created by the author to illustrate medical situations.

Acknowledgments

I would like to acknowledge the people who were most important during the writing of this book. First and foremost, I would like to thank my editors Kerry Smith and Katrina Schroeder for their wisdom, guidance, and support during this project. Thank you to Barbara Doyen for bringing the project to me. I am also very appreciative of the expertise offered by rheumatologist Scott J. Zashin, M.D.

On a more personal level, I thank my mother for her ever-present love, care, and concern, especially when I was first diagnosed with rheumatoid arthritis as a teenager. Thanks to everyone in my family for their love and support, and to my husband Rick for love, inspiration, and making me better than I am alone.

I am very grateful to the doctors and surgeons who help manage my disease, and for the friends I have met in person and online who help inspire me and others who live with arthritis. And finally, thank you to my brother John, who for a lifetime has made me believe I could do it.

Contents

Introduction

IT CAN BE COMPLETELY UNNERVING to have nothing wrong with you one day and severe pain the next day. Since pain is a somewhat common symptom associated with many different conditions, it is hard to know initially what to do or how to react to the sudden change. Not every type of arthritis develops suddenly, but that sense of confusion that builds when you accept that it's not going to go away can sometimes lead you down the wrong path.

No matter what type of arthritis you have, early diagnosis and early treatment can help prevent joint damage and disability. There are many approaches to treating arthritis, both conventional and alternative. There are myriad books written on the subject. The Internet provides even more information about arthritis. It can almost be considered too much information, because a person experiencing the initial onset of arthritis symptoms often doesn't know where to begin. Should you pick up a book about osteoarthritis and learn all about it? Maybe you should choose the book about rheumatoid arthritis? Perhaps it's sufficient to self-treat with over-the-counter arthritis medications? How do you know you are making the right decisions?

Choosing the right starting point can impact the course of your disease. It's imperative to be evaluated by a rheumatologist, a specialist in diagnosing and treating arthritis and related conditions. Getting an accurate diagnosis is the first step to getting proper treatment and managing the disease.

We know for sure that it is important for you to be a partner in your own health care and actively participate in the decision-making process. In this book, we offer basic information about the most common types of arthritis. We guide you through the diagnostic process and make sure you know what to expect from your doctor or rheumatologist. We advise you about the questions you should be asking.

There is also an extensive section on treatment options and information about the benefits and risks associated with arthritis treatments. Throughout the book, there is practical advice that will help you cope with the physical, emotional, and financial impact of living with arthritis. There is important information that sorts out the myths and misconceptions about arthritis from the facts you need to know. You'll also take a peek at the future and consider how arthritis research is helping you today and how it will help you in the years ahead. We also let you know how you can become an advocate for arthritis research.

Chronic arthritis affects every aspect of daily living. This practical guide will show you how to live better with arthritis. The day you are diagnosed with arthritis is the first day of your new reality. Your new reality can overwhelm you, or you can choose to face it with courage and perseverance. Your willingness to accept your new reality and adjust and adapt to it, as well as your ability to cope and an unwillingness to give up, are all factors that will influence how well you live with arthritis.

The intent of this book is to help you learn about the disease, teach you to be your own advocate, help you make better decisions, and inspire you to realize that there is still a high quality of life after an arthritis diagnosis. The first step: Understanding that change is inevitable.

CHAPTER 1

Basic Facts about Arthritis

YOU'VE PROBABLY SEEN advertisements pitching over-the-counter medications to treat "minor arthritis pain." The ads can give a false impression and foster misconceptions about arthritis. Patients may believe the disease is no big deal and delay going to the doctor for an accurate diagnosis and treatment that can prevent joint damage and disability. Being informed and learning about arthritis will help you make better decisions and guide you toward better health care.

What Is Arthritis?

Arthritis literally means "joint inflammation." *Arthr* refers to the joints and *itis* means inflammation; yet it's much more complicated than that. Arthritis is not a single disease; it is a broad term for many conditions that affect the joints, muscles, and tendons. Some arthritic conditions can have systemic effects as well, affecting the skin and other organs.

There are over 100 different types of arthritis, but about 10 percent of those are considered common, leaving a handful to account for the majority of arthritis cases. Certain types of arthritis can be difficult to diagnose, so it's important for you to be evaluated by a doctor to ensure an accurate diagnosis of your condition. Your treatment regimen depends on an accurate diagnosis, and early diagnosis and treatment are imperative for controlling symptoms and managing the disease.

The medical term *arthritis* is commonly used for what are actually *rheumatic diseases*. The two terms are used interchangeably, though there is a technical difference. *Rheumatism*, a third term, is somewhat old-fashioned, but is sometimes used interchangeably with *arthritis* and *rheumatic disease.*

Alert

Most types of arthritis are chronic, meaning they last a long time, as opposed to acute conditions, which are of brief duration. Symptoms of arthritis may flare in an acute pattern, but the disease itself is chronic and lasts a lifetime for most afflicted people.

Rheumatic Disease

Rheumatic disease refers to conditions that primarily affect the joints of the body and supporting structures, including tendons, ligaments, muscles, and bones. The primary characteristics of rheumatic diseases include inflammation and loss of function in one or more connective/supportive structures within the body. Internal organs can also be affected by rheumatic disease. Some rheumatic diseases are connective tissue diseases, while others are considered autoimmune diseases.

Rheumatism

Rheumatism is mostly seen in medical history or old medical texts. In everyday language, it is not used that much. It is appropriate to use the terms *rheumatism* and *rheumatic diseases* interchangeably—they are synonymous.

Rheumatism is further divided according to the location and characteristics of symptoms (e.g. localized rheumatism, regional rheumatism, generalized rheumatism).

Arthritis

Arthritis can be likened to a subset of the rheumatic diseases. Arthritis is characterized by joint pain, joint stiffness, joint inflammation, joint damage, and in some cases joint deformity. For example, lupus is a rheumatic disease that is also considered an autoimmune disease involving the organs and joints. Because joint pain and joint inflammation are prominent characteristics of lupus, the disease is considered a type of arthritis, as well as a rheumatic disease.

Going forward, you will learn more about arthritis in general and the different types of arthritis. You will learn how their symptoms can overlap, making diagnosis sometimes difficult. You will learn about the common types of arthritis and some of the less common types.

Be open to learning as much as you possibly can about arthritis. According to research from the National Institute of Arthritis and Musculoskeletal and Skin Diseases (NIAMS), patients who are well informed and actively participate in their own health care have less pain and make fewer visits to the doctor.

Before learning anything else about arthritis, many people want to know up front if there is a cure for the disease. The short answer: There is no cure for arthritis.

Recognizing the symptoms, knowing when to see a doctor, being compliant with treatment, and never giving up are important patient goals. Learning about osteoarthritis, rheumatoid arthritis, juvenile rheumatoid arthritis, psoriatic arthritis, ankylosing spondylitis, and other types of arthritis will help you recognize overlapping symptoms between the conditions and learn what characteristics distinguish one condition from another. Ultimately, what you, as an arthritis patient, need to focus on should become clearer.

Arthritis Signs and Symptoms

The various types of arthritis have different symptoms. Common arthritis symptoms include:

- Swelling in one or more joints
- Joint stiffness (Inflammatory arthritis may be associated with forty-five minutes or more of stiffness, but noninflammatory arthritis is still associated with morning stiffness that may last less than thirty minutes.)
- Persistent or recurring pain or tenderness in a joint

- Difficulty using or moving a joint (i.e. loss of function, loss of normal range of motion)
- Warmth and redness in or around a joint, indicative of inflammation

Beyond those common symptoms of arthritis, patients can experience joint deformity, crepitus (cracking sound or grating feeling in the joints), fever, unexplained weight loss, severe fatigue, weakness, and malaise (vague feeling of discomfort). Specific symptoms, including where or how they are manifested, are associated with specific types of arthritis.

Essential

Symptoms of arthritis can develop suddenly or gradually. Similarly, progression of the disease can be fast and furious, or slow and seemingly uneventful, especially at first. No two cases of arthritis are alike, at disease onset or years after disease onset.

The next chapter covers common types of arthritis and delves into symptoms associated with specific types of arthritis. The emphasis on getting an accurate diagnosis and early treatment, both of which are discussed in subsequent chapters, will become evident.

Recognizing Joint Problems

If you suspect you have arthritis, you must have noticed a change in how you feel or how you can do certain things. You can do a self-test, which will point out your problems and allow you to gather information for when you do go to the doctor for the first time. Ask yourself these questions:

- Has climbing stairs become more difficult?
- Do you experience hip or knee pain when walking two or more blocks?

- Do you have pain and stiffness in one or both of your hands on a daily basis?
- Do you have problems when brushing your hair?
- Do you have some difficulty when getting dressed in the morning?
- Do you have problems getting on or off of a normal toilet?
- Do you have difficulty getting up from a straight-backed chair that has no arms?
- Do you have difficulty getting in or out of a car?
- Do you have any other functional limitations that developed recently?

Arthritis Risk Factors

Certain risk factors can increase the likelihood that you may develop arthritis. As you consider the signs and symptoms of arthritis, as well as any functional limitations you have noticed, also consider whether you have any of the known risk factors for arthritis.

- Age—Though you can develop arthritis at any age, generally, the risk of developing the disease increases with age.
- Gender—Sixty percent of people with arthritis are women. Most types of arthritis, but not all, are more common in women.
- Genetics—The presence of specific genes increases the risk of developing certain types of arthritis.
- Obesity—Excess weight has been associated with an increased risk of arthritis in weight-bearing joints.
- Joint injury—Trauma to a joint can increase the risk of developing arthritis in that joint.
- Infection—An infection in a joint can lead to arthritis in the affected joint.
- Occupation—Jobs that involve repetitive motions may increase the risk of arthritis in the affected joints.
- Smoking—Smoking has been associated with an increased risk of developing rheumatoid arthritis.

- Family history—A family history of arthritis is considered a risk factor for developing arthritis.

According to the Centers for Disease Control (CDC), some of the risk factors for arthritis are modifiable; other risk factors are not. If you can modify one or more of the factors, you may be able to lower your risk for developing arthritis.

Arthritis Is Not a Single Disease

You have been diagnosed with arthritis, but the diagnostic process does not stop there. Your doctor will also need to determine what type of arthritis you have. It's important to know the specific type of arthritis because each type has different treatment options. Some types of arthritis are divided further into subtypes. Using juvenile rheumatoid arthritis (JRA) as an example, JRA is one of more than 100 types of arthritis. There isn't only one type of juvenile rheumatoid arthritis, however; there are six recognized types.

The American College of Rheumatology (*www.rheumatology. org*) offers criteria for the classification of the different types of arthritis. Also, the pattern of affected joints can help differentiate between these three types of arthritis:

- Monoarthritis—arthritis in a single joint
- Polyarthritis—arthritis in many joints
- Oligoarthritis—arthritis in a few joints (no more than six)

Joint symptoms can occur alone or in combination with other symptoms. Characteristic patterns of joint symptoms can distinguish between inflammatory and noninflammatory types of arthritis. Characteristically, inflammatory types of arthritis produce joint pain and joint stiffness following a period of rest. Noninflammatory types of arthritis exhibit symptoms provoked by movement and weight-bearing activity, which calm after a period of rest. Joint symptoms associated with inflammatory types of arthritis often occur in a symmetrical pattern (for example, both knees), while joint symptoms associated with noninflammatory types of arthritis are typically non-symmetrical (for example, one knee).

Fact

Not only are there more than 100 types of arthritis, an individual patient can have more than one type of arthritis simultaneously. For example, a rheumatoid arthritis patient can also have osteoarthritis, fibromyalgia, or gout.

Other symptoms that accompany joint symptoms can provide more clues, leading to a specific diagnosis. If any of the following symptoms accompany joint symptoms, it may serve as combined, useful diagnostic evidence:

- Muscle weakness
- Severe or persistent fatigue
- Rash
- Hair loss
- Mouth or nose ulcers
- Chest pains
- Hands or feet that change colors with cold weather (e.g. white followed by blue discoloration)
- Dry eyes or mouth
- Night sweats
- Skin abnormalities or nodules
- Sleep problems
- Other comorbid conditions (two or more conditions that occur together)

Saying that you have arthritis is a very general statement. Media advertisements for a medication to treat "minor arthritis pain" are irrelevant. Such generalities and vague statements have little value and detract from the reality of arthritis, which is that there are many types of arthritis and a patient is not always quickly or easily diagnosed. Proper treatment can even be delayed, because diagnosing arthritis is a process, and can sometimes be a very long one.

Misconceptions and misunderstandings about arthritis also detract from the reality of arthritis. Learning about your disease will help you educate and enlighten others about arthritis. People who don't understand the disease make the plight of people living with arthritis worse. Promoting more awareness about arthritis is essential.

Misconceptions about Arthritis

Aside from the misconception that arthritis is a minor inconvenience, there are other common misconceptions associated with the disease. It is curious that the common myths and misconceptions about arthritis have persisted throughout so many years.

One common misconception is that arthritis is just an old person's disease. Other misconceptions have to do with cold weather, poor diet, the "cure," and the variability of symptoms from day to day or hour to hour. Sorting arthritis myths from facts can be tricky.

Imperfect climate is not the cause of arthritis. It is true that some arthritis patients feel better in warm climates rather than cold climates. The warmth makes arthritis symptoms feel better. Just as climate is not the cause, it also is not the cure for arthritis. If it were, there would be no people with arthritis living in cold climates.

Question

Is arthritis only a disease of older persons?
Arthritis is not just an old person's disease. People of any age can develop arthritis, including children. Certain types of arthritis (e.g., osteoarthritis) are more common among older persons, but not exclusive to older persons.

Poor diet does not cause arthritis. There is no scientific evidence supporting the theory that diet causes arthritis, though there are a couple of exceptions. Gout is affected by a high-purine diet. Purines are part of all human tissue and are found in many foods. Uric acid results from the breakdown of purines, and excess uric acid causes gout. Also, food allergies can produce arthritis-like symptoms. And though people are still advised to eat a healthy, balanced diet, a good diet doesn't cure arthritis.

L. Essential

Joint replacements are not only for older persons with arthritis. Pain and quality of life are the factors that should decide when you are ready to have a joint replacement. The decision is not age-dependent. Many young people with arthritis successfully have joint replacement surgery.

Researchers have made progress with regard to developing better treatments and in some cases slowing disease progression and preventing joint deformity, but so far there is no cure. It is important for people to know there is no cure for arthritis because unproven remedies often tout a cure. Don't be misled.

The duration and severity of arthritis symptoms can be variable. Arthritis symptoms can vary between two arthritis patients or from one day to the next for the same patient. It's not possible to compare. Arthritis is inconsistent and contradictory at times. Fatigue and pain may be better or worse on any given day. The nature of arthritis is that it doesn't stay the same.

Limitations imposed by arthritis may restrict what you can do, but it doesn't mean you can't do anything. It's wrong to view a person as totally dependent when she isn't. People with arthritis may need help with some things, but they can still do a lot for themselves. Some people misunderstand this and and are overprotective, thinking your condition is worse than it is.

Misconceptions persist despite more information and better information being within your grasp. As you go through the book, the misconceptions should fade away and you should remember the true facts about arthritis.

The Prevalence of Arthritis

According to the Centers for Disease Control and Prevention (CDC), arthritis is highly prevalent among adults in the United States. The CDC also points out that arthritis is the nation's leading cause of disability and is associated with substantial activity limitation, work disability, reduced quality of life, and high health-care costs.

The latest statistics from the CDC indicate that an estimated 46 million adults in the United States reported being told by a doctor that they have some form of arthritis, rheumatoid arthritis, gout, lupus, or fibromyalgia. Doctor-diagnosed arthritis was reported by 21 percent, or 1 in 5, of adults in the United States. In 2002, 51 percent of adults seventy-five years old and over reported having received a diagnosis of arthritis.

There are 25.9 million women with doctor-diagnosed arthritis, while 16.8 million men have doctor-diagnosed arthritis. According to the CDC:

- Approximately 21 million adults have osteoarthritis.
- About 2.1 million adults have rheumatoid arthritis.
- About 5.1 million adults report doctor-diagnosed gout.
- An estimated 3.7 million adults have fibromyalgia.

Prevalence statistics according to age revealed that:

- Approximately 300,000 children under seventeen years old have juvenile arthritis.
- 7.9 percent (8.5 million) of people eighteen to forty-four years old have doctor-diagnosed arthritis.
- 28.8 percent (18.5 million) of people forty-five to sixty-four years old have doctor-diagnosed arthritis.
- 47.8 percent (15.7 million) of people sixty-five and over report having doctor-diagnosed arthritis.

As you may expect, people who report doctor-diagnosed arthritis have significantly worse Health Related Quality of Life measures than people without arthritis, twice as many unhealthy days, and three times as many activity limitations than people who do not have arthritis.

The prevalence statistics are striking. According to the Arthritis Foundation, about 80 percent of adults have arthritis or know someone who has arthritis. Though the disease is often associated with an aging population, it is important to remember that statistics show 68 percent of people with arthritis or chronic joint symptoms are under sixty-five years old.

Who Can Get Arthritis?

Anyone can get arthritis. Men, women, and children can develop the chronic disease. Some types of arthritis are more common in women, while other types are more common in men. Some types of arthritis are more prevalent in certain racial or ethnic groups.

Of the people reporting doctor-diagnosed arthritis, 34 million were Caucasian, 2.6 million were Hispanic adults, and 4.5 million were African Americans.

With the expectation that the prevalence of arthritis will rise as the baby-boomer generation ages, it is important to be aware of risk factors. For example, it's important to maintain your ideal weight to lower your risk of developing arthritis. The CDC reports that 66 percent of adults with doctor-diagnosed arthritis are overweight or obese, compared to 53 percent of adults without doctor-diagnosed arthritis.

Besides women, older adults, and those who are overweight, people with little education and people who are physically inactive have a higher prevalence of arthritis. The high prevalence of arthritis across all demographic groups points out the need for greater awareness of risk factors and symptom management so arthritis-attributable activity limitations and disability can be reduced. Modifiable risk factors should get particular attention. Gender is not a modifiable risk factor, but weight, smoking, and activity level are examples of modifiable risk factors.

Fact

Approximately 15 percent of underweight adults report having doctor-diagnosed arthritis, compared to 17.5 percent of those who are normal weight, 21 percent who are overweight, and 31 percent of Americans who are obese.

With the availability of several new arthritis treatments in the past decade and researchers focused on improving the outlook for arthritis patients, quality of life should improve with proper care and intervention. Reducing pain, preventing disability, and improving function are the goals for patients who live with arthritis. It begins with learning about the disease and learning how you can help yourself.

Chapter 2

Common Types of Arthritis

THOUGH THE NAME SEEMS REPRESENTATIVE of a single disease, arthritis is actually a group of diseases that have symptoms affecting the joints of the body and the tissues that surround the joints. Over 100 different types of arthritis range from mild forms of the disease to types that can be severe and disabling. Some types are rare, while about a dozen are considered common types of arthritis.

Osteoarthritis

Osteoarthritis is the most common type of arthritis. It is the type of arthritis most people are familiar with because it is most prevalent and is associated with aging. Osteoarthritis is also known by other names that are more reflective of the underlying disease process, including: "wear-and-tear" arthritis, degenerative arthritis, degenerative joint disease, and osteoarthrosis.

In a healthy person, the ends of the bones that form a joint are cushioned by cartilage, allowing for smooth, unconstrained movement of the joint. With osteoarthritis, the cartilage breaks down and deteriorates. As the cartilage deteriorates and is worn away, bone rubs on bone, resulting in pain, stiffness, and reduced mobility.

Bone spurs (also known as osteophytes) may develop which intrude on the joint space and fragments of bone may dislodge, which also interferes with normal movement of the joint. The lining of the joint, or synovium, becomes inflamed as cartilage breaks down, starting a process which itself causes even more cartilage deterioration and joint damage.

Symptoms of Osteoarthritis

Osteoarthritis can affect any joint, but the weight-bearing joints of the hips, knees, and spine are most commonly symptomatic. It is also not unusual for osteoarthritis to develop in the joints of the fingers or feet. A single joint or multiple joints may be affected by osteoarthritis.

 Alert

According to the Arthritis Foundation, osteoarthritis of the knees and hips is the most common cause of arthritis-related disability in the United States. In people who have knee osteoarthritis, moderate physical activity at least three times per week can reduce the risk of arthritis-related disability by 47 percent.

Signs and symptoms associated with osteoarthritis include:

- Gradual onset of symptoms
- Joint stiffness in the morning, which usually lasts less than one half hour
- Joint stiffness following inactivity or staying in one position for a prolonged period
- Joint pain or stiffness following overuse of the affected joint
- Joint pain that is typically worse in the evening than the morning
- Limited range of motion in the affected joint
- Joints that lock up or feel like they are giving out
- Localized inflammation
- Bony outgrowths
- Crepitus (a crackling noise)

Diagnosis and Treatment of Osteoarthritis

X-ray evidence of joint damage, a physical examination performed by your doctor, and a medical history that includes details about the onset of symptoms help diagnose osteoarthritis. Blood tests are ordered for the purpose of ruling out other types of arthritis. For example, blood test results that are abnormal in rheumatoid arthritis or other inflammatory forms of arthritis are usually normal in cases of osteoarthritis.

Though there is no cure for osteoarthritis, treatment is aimed at controlling symptoms, preserving residual joint function, and improving mobility. Medications are commonly prescribed to treat osteoarthritis (for example, NSAIDs and analgesics). Local injections of corticosteroids or viscosupplementation agents are also treatment options.

Some osteoarthritis patients find relief from topical creams or certain nutritional supplements. You may find that hot or cold packs can relieve symptoms. The benefits of exercise, physical therapy, and weight management can't be understated for controlling pain and symptoms associated with osteoarthritis. Surgery, though considered a last-resort treatment option for severe cases, can yield dramatic results.

Risk Factors and Prevalence of Osteoarthritis

Risk factors for osteoarthritis include age, gender, heredity, and obesity. Other risk factors may include previous injury, developmental abnormalities, and occupation.

Approximately 21 million Americans have been diagnosed with osteoarthritis. Though osteoarthritis can affect people of any age, it is more prevalent among older people. If x-rays were taken of everyone over seventy years old, about 70 percent would reveal x-ray evidence of osteoarthritis. Interestingly, only half of the group with x-ray evidence actually becomes symptomatic.

In general, more women than men develop osteoarthritis. However, under the age of fifty-five, more men than women are likely to develop osteoarthritis.

Obesity, because of the additional stress added to weight-bearing joints, is a risk factor for developing osteoarthritis. The knee joint is most affected by osteoarthritis in people carrying excess weight. Being mindful of the risk factors, especially those you can control such as your weight, may impact the course of your disease.

Fact

> According to the CDC, weight loss of eleven pounds reduces the risk of developing knee osteoarthritis by 50 percent. One study from the Parker Institute concluded that in patients with knee osteoarthritis, weight reduction of 10 percent improved function by 28 percent.

Rheumatoid Arthritis

Rheumatoid arthritis is an autoimmune, systemic, inflammatory form of arthritis. It is a chronic, progressive disease. Joints are the main part of the body affected by rheumatoid arthritis, but systemic involvement is possible too, meaning that organs can be affected.

Joint damage develops differently in rheumatoid arthritis than osteoarthritis. With rheumatoid arthritis, immune cells go awry and attack the body's own healthy tissues. This happens when a three-phase inflammatory process takes place: Swelling of the joint lining (synovium) occurs; pannus (inflamed tissue spreads from the synovial membrane and invades the joint) causes the synovium to thicken; and inflamed cells release enzymes which can digest bone and cartilage, resulting in joint damage.

Symptoms of Rheumatoid Arthritis

As with osteoarthritis, rheumatoid arthritis can affect any joint. A major difference between the two most common forms of arthritis is that rheumatoid arthritis usually affects joints symmetrically. With rheumatoid arthritis, it is common for the same joint on both sides of the body to be affected (e.g., if your left knee is affected, your right knee will likely be affected too).

Rheumatoid arthritis causes joint pain, stiffness, swelling, redness, warmth, and limited range of motion. Damage can occur to tendons and ligaments, as well as bone and cartilage. Other signs and symptoms that point to rheumatoid arthritis include:

- Prolonged morning stiffness that lasts more than an hour
- Small joints of hands and feet commonly affected
- Malaise (a vague feeling of discomfort)
- Fatigue
- Low-grade fever
- Loss of appetite
- Rheumatoid nodules (a small collection or growth of tissue)
- Pain associated with prolonged sitting or staying in one position
- An association with Sjögren's syndrome (dry eyes and mouth)

Symptoms associated with rheumatoid arthritis are variable; the course of disease is not exactly alike for any two rheumatoid arthritis patients. Your individual course of disease may vary as well, as you experience periods of flares and remissions.

Diagnosis and Treatment of Rheumatoid Arthritis

Once again, there is no single test used to definitively diagnose rheumatoid arthritis. Other types of arthritis have similar symptoms, making rheumatoid arthritis difficult to diagnose. There are a number of diagnostic tools and factors that, used in combination, help formulate the diagnosis. A medical history and physical examination are used initially to search for symptoms.

Laboratory blood tests can reveal abnormalities consistent with having rheumatoid arthritis. Rheumatoid factor, erythrocyte sedimentation rate, C-reactive protein, and anti-CCP tests are routinely ordered to help diagnose rheumatoid arthritis. X-rays and MRIs (magnetic resonance imaging) are useful for showing evidence of joint damage. In the first few months after onset of the disease the evidence may not yet appear on x-ray images.

Early diagnosis is important so that treatment can begin. Decades ago, rheumatoid arthritis was treated conservatively. Conventional thinking was that patients should be treated with the least amount of medication that evoked a response. With the development of newer medications, some of which have the potential to slow disease progression and prevent severe joint erosions, researchers and the medical community agree that early, aggressive treatment is the way to go for patients who have no contraindications (i.e., reasons a patient should not take a particular medication).

Alert

> Early aggressive treatment is emphasized for rheumatoid arthritis because joint damage often occurs within the first two years of the disease. People with rheumatoid arthritis have a high risk of disability and twice the risk of mortality as people in the general population who do not have the disease.

There is no cure for rheumatoid arthritis, but treatment can help control symptoms and preserve joint function. Medications, along with other complementary treatments, are usually considered the best course of treatment for most rheumatoid arthritis patients. There are several medications used to treat rheumatoid arthritis, which you will read about in a later chapter. It is not uncommon for patients to try several treatments before deciding which ones yield optimum results. You may have to make changes to your treatment plan several times over the course of months and years.

Risk Factors and Prevalence of Rheumatoid Arthritis

Numerous studies have looked at what causes the abnormal immune response associated with rheumatoid arthritis. Genetic predisposition combined with a triggering event is a popular theory.

Rheumatoid arthritis can affect anyone of any age, including children. Typically, the age of onset for rheumatoid arthritis is between thirty and sixty years of age. Approximately 2.1 million people in the United States are affected by rheumatoid arthritis (about 1 percent–2 percent worldwide). About 70 to 75 percent of rheumatoid arthritis patients are women. Of lifestyle factors, smoking has been shown to increase the risk of developing rheumatoid arthritis.

Psoriatic Arthritis

Psoriatic arthritis is a type of arthritis belonging to the group known as the spondyloarthropathies. Psoriatic arthritis, as its name indicates, combines aspects of chronic joint pain and the skin disease psoriasis. Like rheumatoid arthritis, psoriatic arthritis is an inflammatory form of arthritis.

In 85 percent of patients who develop psoriatic arthritis, symptoms of psoriasis appear before symptoms of arthritis, or at the same time. In up to 15 percent of cases, arthritis precedes symptoms of psoriasis.

Symptoms of Psoriatic Arthritis

There are five types of psoriatic arthritis categorized by symptoms:

- Symmetric
- Asymmetric
- Distal interphalangeal predominant
- Spondylitis
- Arthritis mutilans

Symmetric psoriatic arthritis affects joints on both sides of the body. It is similar to rheumatoid arthritis because it affects multiple joints, but is generally considered milder than rheumatoid arthritis. With psoriatic arthritis there is usually less deformity than is characteristic of rheumatoid arthritis.

Asymmetric psoriatic arthritis can affect any joint of the body, but not the same joint on both sides of the body, as is the case with the symmetric type. Sausage-like toes and fingers from swelling are common characteristics of asymmetric psoriatic arthritis. Asymmetric is considered the most common type of psoriatic arthritis.

Distal interphalangeal predominant psoriatic arthritis primarily involves the distal joints of the fingers and toes. Nail changes are also a predominant feature.

Spondylitis psoriatic arthritis is characterized by inflammation of the spine. About half of the patients with the spondylitis type have a genetic marker, HLA-B27.

Arthritis mutilans is a very rare, but severe and disabling type of psoriatic arthritis. Joint deformity is the primary symptom, with small joints in the hands and feet most affected. Neck and lower-back pain are also problematic.

Question

Is psoriasis a contagious skin condition?
Psoriasis is not contagious. Psoriatic lesions appear as whitish, scaly patches of inflamed cells, but the lesions are not infectious and are not open wounds.

Diagnosis and Treatment of Psoriatic Arthritis

As with the other types of arthritis already mentioned, a medical history and physical examination are important during the diagnostic process. Blood tests are ordered, but with the intent of ruling out other types of arthritis. The erythrocyte sedimentation rate that is often elevated with rheumatoid arthritis may also be elevated with psoriatic arthritis. Elevated levels of blood uric acid are not uncommon, making it necessary to rule out gout.

The medications used to treat psoriatic arthritis are basically the same as those used to treat rheumatoid arthritis. Additionally, topical creams and light treatments help with the psoriasis.

Risk Factors and Prevalence of Psoriatic Arthritis

Men and women are affected equally by psoriatic arthritis. The disease usually has an age of onset between thirty and fifty years old. About 15 percent of psoriasis sufferers go on to develop psoriatic arthritis. Estimates suggest that 40 percent of people with psoriatic arthritis have a family history of psoriasis or arthritis, pointing to a genetic component. About 1 million Americans have psoriatic arthritis. About 2 percent of Caucasian people in North America suffer with psoriasis.

Juvenile Rheumatoid Arthritis (JRA)

About 300,000 children in America are affected by some form of juvenile arthritis or rheumatic disease. Joint inflammation and joint stiffness which persist for more than six weeks in a child age sixteen years old or younger is the initial criteria used to diagnose juvenile rheumatoid arthritis, more commonly referred to as JRA. There are three classifications for juvenile rheumatoid arthritis: pauciarticular, polyarticular, and systemic.

Pauciarticular JRA

Pauciarticular JRA affects four or fewer joints. About 50 percent of children with JRA have the pauciarticular type, making it the most common type of JRA. This type is further subdivided into early onset and late onset. Early onset affects more girls than boys by a 4:1 ratio. Typically, the children are very young, under five years of age. A common symptom associated with pauciarticular JRA is inflammation of the eye. Late onset is more common in boys, half of whom are positive for genetic marker HLA-B27. The large joints are commonly affected, and if there is eye inflammation it is usually not chronic.

Polyarticular JRA

Polyarticular JRA affects five or more joints and affects about 30 to 40 percent of children who have JRA. Girls are affected more often than boys by a 3:1 ratio. The small joints are more commonly affected, but large joints can also be affected. Two sub-groups of polyarticular JRA are determined by the presence or absence of rheumatoid factor. Most polyarticular JRA patients who are positive for rheumatoid factor are girls, age eight years old or older with symmetric arthritis affecting the small joints, who are also positive for HLA-DR4 (a genetic factor). They typically have a more severe course of the disease that resembles adult rheumatoid arthritis.

Systemic JRA

Systemic JRA, also referred to as Still's disease, equally affects boys and girls, with a usual age of onset between one and six years old. Approximately 10 percent of children with JRA have the systemic type. Fever and skin rash are distinguishing features. Internal organs may be affected. Usually the child is negative for rheumatoid factor and antinuclear antibodies.

L. Essential

The American Juvenile Arthritis Organization (AJAO) is a valuable resource for children, teens, and young adults affected by juvenile arthritis. AJAO, a council of the Arthritis Foundation, provides information, programs, and support for JRA patients and their families. The Web site can be found at ⌁*www.arthritis .org/communities/juvenile_arthritis/about_ajao.asp.*

Juvenile Arthritis—Naming Issues

It has been suggested that the term *juvenile rheumatoid arthritis* is confusing because it implies it's the same condition as adult rheumatoid arthritis, just with earlier onset. However, most children with arthritis do not have a form of disease that correlates with adult-onset rheumatoid arthritis. To make the distinction, some resources refer to childhood arthritis as juvenile chronic arthritis (JCA) or juvenile idiopathic arthritis (JIA). Still others suggest that simply juvenile arthritis (JA) is more accurate. Still, because old habits die hard, *juvenile rheumatoid arthritis* remains a commonly used terminology. It is important to remember that juvenile arthritis is not a single disease; it refers to a group of symptoms with many causes.

Young children may not complain of pain, so parents must be observant of signs that could be indicative of arthritis. Signs may include fatigue, lack of appetite, and lack of interest in playing or activities that would normally elicit a positive response. If the child is old enough to walk, the parent may also observe a subtle limp. A pediatrician or family doctor should be consulted. The signs and symptoms shouldn't be shrugged off as growing pains. If needed, a consultation with a pediatric rheumatologist may be ordered. Early diagnosis and treatment is very important so symptoms can be managed.

Ankylosing Spondylitis

In the United States, about 129 out of 100,000 people have ankylosing spondylitis. Ankylosing spondylitis (previously referred to as rheumatoid spondylitis, Marie-Strumpell's spondylitis, and poker back) is a chronic inflammatory type of arthritis that primarily affects the sacroiliac joints and the spine. The lower back is most often affected, but the mid-portion of the back and neck can also be involved. Progressive stiffening of the spine is common, and ankylosis (fusion) of some or all of the spinal joints occurs in later years for many but not all patients. There is a concern about fusion occurring in a non-upright position. Good posture, as well as early treatment, is important.

Joints other than the spinal joints can also be involved. The hips, knees, and shoulders may be involved; however, it is uncommon for the small joints of the hands and feet, wrists, or ankles to be affected by ankylosing spondylitis.

Ankylosing spondylitis is classified as one of the spondyloarthropathies because of shared characteristics with psoriatic arthritis and reactive arthritis. According to the Primer on Rheumatic Diseases (Arthritis Foundation), there is a strong inherited component associated with ankylosing spondylitis. About 90 percent of people with ankylosing spondylitis have the genetic marker HLA-B27. The test for the genetic marker is not definitive for ankylosing spondylitis, but suggests a predisposition to it. Many people with ankylosing spondylitis have family members with the disease. About 6 percent of the general population has the genetic marker as well, but will likely not develop ankylosing spondylitis.

Early diagnosis is important, but it is not uncommon for the diagnosis to come with some difficulty. X-ray evidence of ankylosing spondylitis may not appear for many years. Recognizing common symptoms so you can tell your doctor what you are experiencing is helpful. Common symptoms include:

- Back pain and stiffness that can result in bent posture
- Back pain that persists for more than three months
- Back pain which is dull as opposed to sharp
- Morning stiffness, especially of the back or spine
- Pain in areas other than the back (e.g., ribs, shoulder blades, hips, thighs, heels)
- Iritis (inflammation of the eye)

Both men and women can develop ankylosing spondylitis, but it is three times more prevalent in men. Onset of the disease is usually between fifteen and forty years old, though it can develop at any age. Treatment options are similar to those used to treat rheumatoid arthritis: medications to control inflammation; physical therapy to maintain mobility and joint flexibility; and surgery to repair joint damage. However, there is no surgery to repair the spine for this disease. Ankylosing spondylitis is usually a slow, progressive disease and symptoms range from mild to severe. Most people with ankylosing spondylitis continue to work and function relatively normally. Long duration of the disease can result in neurological, cardiac, and pulmonary complications, but such complications are very rare.

Alert

Maintaining good posture is very important for people with ankylosing spondylitis. Make sure to keep your spine straight when walking or sitting. It is best to sleep on a firm mattress or to sleep on your stomach, with either a thin pillow or no pillow. You should refrain from curling up in bed.

Infectious Arthritis

Primary symptoms of infectious arthritis include joint pain and swelling. Usually only one joint is affected, but two or even three joints can be affected. A germ, whether a bacterium, virus, or fungus, is responsible for the inflammation associated with infectious arthritis.

Infectious arthritis can affect people at any age, and affects men and women equally. People with conditions that make it hard to fight infection (for example, diabetes, AIDS, kidney disease) may be more prone to develop infectious arthritis than others. Also, patients with a history of arthritis are more likely to develop infectious arthritis.

Germs have a tendency to infect weak or damaged joints. Patients who have had joint replacements are also more likely to develop infectious arthritis, as germs may target the joint prostheses.

Some of the medications used to treat inflammatory forms of arthritis lower the body's immunity or resistance to infection. If you take these medications, you are more susceptible to developing infection and infectious arthritis. People who work at certain jobs that require the handling of infectious materials may also be more at risk for developing infectious arthritis.

Warning signs for infectious arthritis depend on the causative germ. If the causative germ is a bacterium, pain and swelling is usually localized and comes on suddenly, possibly with fever and chills. If the causative germ is a virus, widespread pain is more common, but with no fever. If the causative germ is a fungus, there is gradual onset of pain and swelling that is either localized or widespread, and mild fever is possible.

The germs have numerous available ports of entry into the body, passing through the skin, nose, throat, ears, or even a wound. The infection itself may make you quite sick before the germ travels to the joints. An infection can be passed from one person to another, but infectious arthritis cannot be passed from one person to another.

Infectious arthritis, due to a bacterium or fungus, has a good chance of being cured if treated early. If treatment is postponed or if treatment is lacking, joint damage can get worse and the infection can spread to other parts of the body.

Medications are usually prescribed to treat inflammation associated with infectious arthritis, and antibiotics or anti-fungal medications are given to treat the infection. There is no medication given to treat a virus.

 Fact

> Most cases of infectious arthritis are caused by bacteria, including gonococcus, staphylococcus, streptococcus, pneumococcus, haemophilus, spirochetes, and tuberculosis. Viruses that can cause infectious arthritis may be associated with infectious hepatitis, mumps, and infectious mononucleosis, but parvovirus is the most common. Fungi are the least-common causative germ of infectious arthritis, but most come from the soil, bird droppings, and plants.

Reactive Arthritis

Reactive arthritis, classified as a seronegative spondyloarthropathy, typically follows an infection. Common causes include food poisoning or another infection of the intestine (called gastrointestinal reactive arthritis). Chlamydia, a sexually transmitted disease, is another common cause of reactive arthritis. Venereal infections of the bladder, urethra, or vagina can also cause reactive arthritis in many patients (called genitourinary or urogenital reactive arthritis). Reactive arthritis itself is not transmittable from one person to another.

Symptoms may include:

- Painful, swollen, stiff joints that may also be red and warm
- Stiffness that may be aggravated in the morning
- Lower-back pain
- Heel pain (such as Achilles heel)
- Eyes sensitive to light
- Mouth sores
- Sores on the genitals

Symptoms typically appear one to three weeks following an intestinal infection. Salmonella, shigella, campylobacter, and yersinia are common causative bacteria associated with intestinal infection. With reactive arthritis, one joint is usually involved rather than multiple joints; it's usually knees, ankles, or toes that are involved. The sacroiliac joints are also commonly involved. Symptoms of reactive arthritis may also affect body parts other than the joints, including tendons, skin, and eyes.

About 50 to 75 percent of patients with reactive arthritis are positive for HLA-B27. The genetic marker points to a genetic predisposition for the disease. Cases of reactive arthritis can resolve in days or weeks, while some take nearly four to twelve months to resolve. Recurring bouts of reactive arthritis are possible. Aside from medications used to treat the infection, anti-inflammatory medications are also used to treat arthritis and joint symptoms.

Reactive arthritis usually affects people between twenty and fifty years old. There is equal prevalence of reactive arthritis among males and females as a result of intestinal infections. However, men are nine times more likely than women to get reactive arthritis following venereal infections.

Question

What is the prognosis for patients who have been diagnosed with reactive arthritis?

According to NIAMS, about 20 percent of people with reactive arthritis will have chronic arthritis symptoms which are mild. Studies have revealed that between 15 and 50 percent of patients will relapse and develop symptoms again sometime after the initial symptoms have resolved. The relapses are possibly associated with reinfection.

Also, according to NIAMS (the National Institute of Arthritis and Musculoskeletal and Skin Diseases), researchers are trying to ascertain more about the causal relationship between infection and reactive arthritis. It's still not known why infection triggers arthritis, and more specifically, why not everyone with an infection develops reactive arthritis. People with HLA-B27 are more at risk for developing reactive arthritis than those who lack the genetic factor, so the answers may, in part, have a genetic basis. Combination treatments, such as antibiotics and TNF blockers or other immunosuppressant medications, are also being studied for treatment of reactive arthritis.

CHAPTER 3

Other Types of Arthritis and Rheumatic Conditions

THERE ARE OTHER ARTHRITIS-RELATED CONDITIONS that aren't considered rare, but are not as common or prevalent as osteoarthritis and rheumatoid arthritis. Some of the less-common types of arthritis can occur as primary diseases or as secondary conditions; it's possible to have more than one type of arthritis. Because of the complexity of each of the conditions and the possibility of overlapping symptoms, it can't be emphasized enough that your doctor must serve as the detective.

Gout and Pseudogout

Gout is recognized as one of the most intensely painful types of arthritis. Pain, inflammation, swelling, warmth, and redness of a single joint are typical symptoms associated with gout. The most common joint affected is the big toe, but other joints can also be affected.

Cause of Gout Versus Cause of Pseudogout

Gout is caused by the accumulation of excess uric acid in the body resulting in the formation of crystals that are deposited in the joints. The deposition of uric acid crystals in the joints causes the inflammatory response. Uric acid is a by-product of the breakdown of purines found in all human tissues and many of the foods you eat. Gout can result from excess production of uric acid in the body or insufficient elimination of uric acid by the kidneys. Gout may be triggered by:

- Eating a diet of purine-rich foods
- Excessive alcohol intake
- Being overweight
- Genetic factors
- Surgery
- The use of certain medications
- Lead exposure
- Joint injury

Pseudogout, as the name implies, is a condition that is often mistaken for gout. A different crystal is involved in pseudogout, however. In pseudogout, calcium pyrophosphate crystals are deposited in the joints. The condition is also referred to as calcium pyrophosphate deposition disease or CPPD. The knees are the most commonly affected joints with pseudogout. Wrists, shoulders, ankles, elbows, or hands can also be affected. Pseudogout may be triggered by:

- Increased age
- Genetic factors
- Hypothyroidism
- Hematochromatosis
- Low magnesium blood levels
- Overactive parathyroid
- Hypercalcemia

Question

Do gout attacks typically come on gradually or occur suddenly?
Gout attacks typically develop very suddenly, and it is common for the first gout episode to occur at night. People can wake with a red, swollen, inflamed toe (or other joint) after going to bed without any signs or symptoms.

Diagnosis and Treatment

The symptoms of gout and pseudogout can be mistaken for other types of inflammatory arthritis. A proper diagnosis comes from identifying the crystal in the fluid of the affected joint. Your doctor will aspirate the fluid from the joint and examine it under a microscope for the presence of the crystals. In gout, the crystals may also be found in tophi, which are deposits found under the skin.

Gout is typically treated with diet modification, weight reduction, adequate fluid intake, and the use of medications that control the inflammation (e.g., NSAIDS or corticosteroids). Other gout medications include: colchicine which treats acute gout attacks, probenecid which helps with elimination of uric acid, and allopurinol which blocks production of uric acid.

Pseudogout is also treated using anti-inflammatory drugs and low doses of colchicine.

Prevalence of Gout

The National Institutes of Health reports that gout accounts for 5 percent of all cases of arthritis. The CDC reports that about 5.1 million adults report having doctor-diagnosed gout.

Anyone can develop gout or pseudogout, but more men than women are affected by gout. Men over the age of forty and women past menopause are at greater risk. Pseudogout crystals are found in about 50 percent of people in their nineties.

Scleroderma

Scleroderma is an arthritis-related condition that is classified as an autoimmune connective-tissue disease. You may think scleroderma is a single disease, but it's not. Scleroderma is a symptom of a group of diseases that are complicated by the abnormal growth of connective tissue supporting skin and other organs. The term *scleroderma* literally means "hard skin." Some types of scleroderma are limited to skin thickening, tightening, and hardening, while other types of scleroderma may affect blood vessels or internal organs.

Scleroderma Types

There are two major types of scleroderma, and those are further classified. The two major types of scleroderma are:

Localized scleroderma—Primarily affects the skin and is further subdivided into morphea and linear. Morphea is characterized by hard, oval patches on the skin. Linear is characterized by a line of thickened, discolored skin commonly on the arms, legs, or forehead.

Systemic sclerosis—Is further subdivided into limited sclero-derma, diffuse scleroderma, and sine scleroderma. Limited scleroderma typically has gradual onset, is limited to certain areas of the body, and may affect internal organs eventually. Diffuse scleroderma is characterized by sudden onset, thickening covering a large area of the body, and may also affect internal organs. Sine scleroderma does not affect the skin.

CREST
Systemic sclerosis patients may have a typical pattern of symptoms referred to as CREST. The acronym CREST stands for:

- Calcinosis—calcium deposits in connective tissue
- Raynaud's phenomenon—small blood-vessel constriction in response to cold or stress
- Esophageal dysfunction—muscle in lower esophagus functions improperly
- Sclerodactyly—tight, thick, shiny skin on toes and fingers
- Telangiectasias—tiny red spots on face and hands

Diagnosing Scleroderma
There is no single test that is used to diagnose scleroderma, although most people with scleroderma are positive for antinuclear antibodies. A physical examination, in combination with blood tests to rule out other conditions, plus telltale symptoms of organ involvement, are all used to formulate a diagnosis.

There is neither a cure for scleroderma, nor a treatment that can prevent the thickening which is characteristic of the disease. While there is no great treatment for the skin, there are reports of benefits with some medications. Medications are usually prescribed for the consequences of scleroderma such as arthritis, pulmonary hypertension, hypertension, heartburn, kidney problems, and more.

Alert

Medications used to treat other autoimmune conditions, including rheumatoid arthritis and lupus, typically have little effect on scleroderma patients. Scleroderma is a somewhat rare disease with only twelve to twenty new cases per million diagnosed each year.

Prevalence of Scleroderma

Approximately 75,000 to 100,000 people in the United States are affected by scleroderma. Women between the ages of thirty and fifty are the most commonly affected group, but men, women, and children can all develop scleroderma.

Lupus

Lupus, short for systemic lupus erythematosus or SLE, is a chronic inflammatory disease that can affect the skin, joints, kidneys, lungs, and nervous system, as well as other organs of the body. Lupus is also considered an autoimmune disease. Common symptoms associated with lupus include:

- Arthritis in multiple joints
- Rashes including the characteristic butterfly-shaped rash over the nose and cheeks
- Fever
- Fatigue
- Weight loss
- Mouth sores or nose sores
- Hair loss
- Seizures or strokes
- Mental issues
- Low blood counts
- Urinalysis showing poor kidney function
- Chest pain or heartburn
- Sun sensitivity

Lupus has other symptoms as well. Some symptoms develop gradually and overlap with symptoms of other conditions, making lupus difficult to diagnose.

There are at least five recognized types of lupus:

Systemic lupus erythematosus—as described previously, this is the type of lupus most often referred to when people speak of lupus

Discoid lupus erythematosus—chronic skin disorder characterized by red, raised rash which appears on the face and scalp typically, but may appear on other areas of the body and may cause scarring. Rash may last and may reoccur. Only a small percentage of people with discoid lupus develop systemic lupus erythematosus

Subacute cutaneous lupus erythematosus—skin lesions on body parts exposed to the sun that do not cause scarring

Drug-induced lupus—a type of lupus caused by medications. Several medications can cause drug-induced lupus, which has symptoms similar to SLE. Symptoms usually go away when the offending medication is completely stopped

Neonatal lupus—a rare form of lupus that can develop in newborn babies of women with systemic lupus erythematosus, Sjögren's syndrome, or even in women who have no disease

Diagnosing and Treating Lupus

A combination of clinical symptoms indicating lupus and blood tests are used to help diagnose lupus.

The presence of antiphospholipid antibodies suggests the possibility of future complications including miscarriage and blood clots.

The course of treatment prescribed for lupus depends on the individual patient's needs. The unpredictability of lupus can make it necessary to change the course of disease treatment at times. NSAIDs, corticosteroids, antimalarial drugs, immunosuppressants, and DMARDs are used to treat lupus.

L. Essential

Nearly all patients with lupus are positive for the antinuclear antibody test. More specific antibody tests, such as anti-double strand DNA (dsDNA) and anti-smith (Sm), are used to confirm the diagnosis of lupus. Complement levels are also useful in diagnosing and monitoring lupus.

Prevalence of Lupus

Lupus affects ten times more women than men. Lupus commonly develops between the ages of eighteen and forty-five, though younger or older people can develop the disease too. African Americans have a higher rate of lupus than other groups. There also appears to be a strong genetic connection. Studies have shown that lupus is more common in families where one family member already has lupus, according to the Arthritis Foundation. According to the CDC, a conservative estimate suggests that lupus affects about 239,000 people in the United States.

Sjögren's Syndrome

Sjögren's syndrome is an inflammatory autoimmune disease that can affect various body parts, but primarily affects the tear and saliva glands, causing dry eyes and dry mouth. People who suffer with dry eyes may be at increased risk for eye infections or damage to the cornea. Patients often complain of eye irritation such as grittiness or a burning sensation. People who have dry mouth may complain of having difficulty swallowing, especially dry foods, and may also have swelling around the face and neck. Dry mouth can increase the risk of dental decay, gingivitis, or oral thrush.

Primary or Secondary Sjögren's Syndrome

The condition is referred to as primary Sjögren's syndrome when there is no other connective-tissue disease associated with it. Sjögren's syndrome may occur commonly in patients with rheumatoid arthritis, and in those cases it is referred to as secondary Sjögren's. Extraglandular complications can occur, but are considered rare, including: joint pain without the presence of another rheumatic disease; rashes from inflammation of small blood vessels, lung, liver, or kidney inflammation; neurological problems (such as numbness and weakness); and malignancy.

Secondary Sjögren's syndrome develops in people who have another rheumatic disease. Most often, the other rheumatic condition is rheumatoid arthritis, lupus, or scleroderma.

Fact

Sjögren's syndrome is named after a Swedish doctor, Henrik Sjögren. Sjögren was the first to describe symptoms of chronic arthritis along with dry eyes and dry mouth in a group of women in the early 1900s. Ninety percent of people with Sjögren's syndrome are women.

Diagnosing and Treating Sjögren's Syndrome

Physical symptoms, blood tests, and special tests are used to diagnose Sjögren's syndrome. The physical symptoms serve as early indicators. Blood tests, such as the antinuclear antibody test and more specific antibody tests for anti-SSA and anti-SSB, are used to confirm the diagnosis. Special tests include the Schirmer test for tear production, salivary gland biopsy, salivary gland scans, and flow testing.

Sjögren's syndrome treatment focuses on relieving the symptoms of dry eyes and dry mouth and includes saliva stimulators, sprays, gels, and gum. Salagen and Evoxac are prescription medications that stimulate the flow of saliva. Dry eyes can be helped with artificial tears or eye ointments, and Restasis or hydroxypropyl cellulose may be prescribed. Extraglandular complications associated with Sjögren's syndrome may be treated with corticosteroids and DMARDs.

For obvious reasons, it is important to consult regularly with a dentist and ophthalmologist as well as your rheumatologist.

Prevalence of Sjögren's Syndrome

Sjögren's syndrome most commonly develops between the ages of forty-five and fifty-five, though it can develop at any age. According to the American College of Rheumatology, ten times more women than men have Sjögren's syndrome, and about half of the affected patients have rheumatoid arthritis or another rheumatic disease. Approximately 1 to 2 percent of the population is affected by Sjögren's syndrome (between 1 and 4 million Americans).

Fibromyalgia

Fibromyalgia is a syndrome which is hard to diagnose and somewhat hard to explain because symptoms can be so variable. Fibromyalgia symptoms primarily include chronic widespread muscular pain, tenderness, and fatigue. Long ago, the disease was called fibrositis, but that was a misnomer because it implied there was inflammation. There is no inflammation associated with the pain and stiffness of the muscles, tendons, and joints seen with fibromyalgia. It is also important to note that fibromyalgia does not affect or damage internal organs.

In 1990, the American College of Rheumatology defined criteria for diagnosing fibromyalgia, which until then wasn't understood very well. The criteria included:

- A history of widespread pain in all four quadrants of the body for three months or longer
- Pain in eleven of eighteen tender points

Fibromyalgia has also been associated with a heightened sensitivity to pain, migratory pain, chronic regional pain, and abnormal central nervous-system function according to some researchers. Other symptoms that are often associated with fibromyalgia include:

- Headaches
- Sleep disturbances
- Irritable bowel or bladder
- Cognitive difficulties (sometimes called fibro fog)
- Jaw pain
- Pelvic pain
- Restless leg syndrome

- Hearing, vision, and balance problems
- Heat and cold sensitivities
- Chemical sensitivities or allergies
- Mitral valve prolapse
- Neurological problems
- Depression or anxiety

Diagnosing and Treating Fibromyalgia

The cause of fibromyalgia is unknown, though there are more and more clues coming from fibromyalgia research. Diagnosis is difficult and is based essentially on symptoms. There are no x-rays, blood tests, or other diagnostic tests available that confirm fibromyalgia.

Fibromyalgia is treated using medication and nonpharmacologic therapies. Medications are chosen based on their ability to relieve symptoms. There is no medication that cures fibromyalgia. Analgesic medications, sleep medications, and antidepressants are often employed to treat fibromyalgia. Guaifenesin, a common cough-syrup ingredient, has been shown to help with fibromyalgia symptoms. Most recently, antiepileptic drugs Neurontin (gabapentin) and Lyrica (pregabalin) have been deemed promising as a treatment for fibromyalgia.

Prevalence of Fibromyalgia

Of people with fibromyalgia, more than 80 percent are women. Most commonly, fibromyalgia strikes between thirty-five and fifty-five years of age. Though men, children, and older persons can also develop fibromyalgia, it is not common in those groups.

Like other rheumatic conditions, fibromyalgia can occur as a primary disease or as a secondary condition along with another rheumatic condition. It has been estimated that fibromyalgia affects between 2 and 4 percent of the population. The CDC estimates that 3.7 million adults in the United States have fibromyalgia.

Alert

> Since pain and tenderness are the primary symptoms of fibro-
> myalgia, it is hard for doctors to set it apart from the other rheu-
> matic diseases that have similar symptoms. X-rays and blood
> tests can be used to rule out other rheumatic conditions, nar-
> rowing the possibilities down to fibromyalgia.

Carpal Tunnel Syndrome

Carpal tunnel syndrome occurs when the median nerve is com-
pressed, resulting in pain, numbness, tingling, weakness, or a burning
sensation in your hand and fingers (except for the little finger, which
remains unaffected). The median nerve runs from your forearm into
your hand through a tunnel in your wrist. Wrist bones comprise the
sides and bottom of the tunnel, while the transverse ligament forms
the top of the tunnel. There are also tendons in the tunnel that con-
nect muscle to bone, but the median nerve is the culprit in carpal
tunnel syndrome. Compression of the median nerve, whether it is
from swelling or narrowing of the tunnel, is the cause of symptoms.
In some cases, enlargement of the median nerve can cause carpal
tunnel syndrome, but more often it is compression of the nerve.

Symptoms associated with carpal tunnel syndrome typically
begin gradually with a sensation of itching, tingling, or burning in the
palm of the hand or index finger, middle fingers, or thumb. One or
both hands may be affected. Often, a feeling of fullness or swelling is
present even when no swelling is truly evident. Clumsiness and problems with tasks requiring manual dexterity are frequent complaints.

Pain may radiate from the hand up to the elbow. It is common for
carpal tunnel symptoms to be worse at night and when the hand is
warm. The muscles at the base of the thumb can atrophy.

Diagnosing and Treating Carpal Tunnel Syndrome

According to the Arthritis Foundation, several physical tests help
diagnose carpal tunnel syndrome. One of the physical tests is called

Tinel's sign; it involves tapping the front of your wrist to check for pain and tingling. Another test, known as Phalen's sign, involves bending the wrist downward, holding, and releasing to check for pain and tingling. Nerve conduction studies can also provide more information. To rule out other conditions, blood tests and x-rays may be ordered.

L. Essential

> The cause of carpal tunnel syndrome is not always known. Wrist injury, swelling associated with different types of arthritis, repetitive motion, certain occupations, diabetes, thyroid disease, inflammatory arthritis such as rheumatoid arthritis, and hormonal changes have all been linked to carpal tunnel syndrome. However, sometimes it can develop for no obvious reason.

Treatment of carpal tunnel syndrome focuses on relieving pain and restoring normal sensations. NSAIDs (nonsteroidal anti–inflammatory drugs) and corticosteroid injections are often used to control inflammation. Protective splints can help the condition from worsening in many cases. If work or certain activities aggravate symptoms, modifying those activities or using adaptive equipment can help by decreasing pain, stiffness, and swelling. Surgery is a common but last-resort solution. The procedure, called a carpal tunnel release, relieves pressure on the median nerve.

Prevalence of Carpal Tunnel Syndrome

Women are more commonly affected by carpal tunnel syndrome than men; according to the National Institutes of Health, women are three times more likely than men to develop carpal tunnel syndrome. Though it can develop at any age, onset is most common after age fifty. Carpal tunnel syndrome is rare in children.

In 2002, the Bureau of Labor Statistics reported that carpal tunnel syndrome accounted for the highest number of missed workdays (twenty-seven), more than missed days due to back injury or broken bones. It has been estimated that about 3 percent of women and 2 percent of men will at some time develop carpal tunnel syndrome.

Lyme Disease

Lyme disease is an infection caused by the spirochete *Borrelia burgdorferi*. The spirochete can live within certain ticks (most commonly the deer tick), and is spread to humans via the bite of an infected tick.

Stages of Lyme Disease

The early localized stage of Lyme disease is characterized by a skin rash (erythema migrans) at the tick-bite site. The rash, which is said to look like a bull's eye, appears anywhere from three days to weeks after the tick bite. Typically, the rash is small at first, but gets larger. If the rash doesn't occur or goes undetected, the bacterium may spread through the bloodstream to other parts of the body. If that happens, the person enters the next stage of Lyme disease, called early disseminated stage, in the weeks after the tick bite.

In the early disseminated stage, the person affected may develop other symptoms including:

- Muscle pain
- Joint pain
- Multiple rashes
- Fever
- Headaches

In late stage infection, which can occur months or years later, there can be more significant arthritis involvement, nervous-system problems, sleep problems, memory issues, and heart problems. Lyme arthritis, as it is sometimes called, typically causes swelling in one or both knees, but it can affect other large joints of the body too.

Diagnosing and Treating Lyme Disease

The CDC has adopted a two-step diagnostic approach for Lyme disease. The ELISA blood test is used to define certain antibodies that would occur as the immune system responds to the infection. The Western blot test is then used to confirm borderline results or positive results. These blood tests shouldn't be performed until the patient shows symptoms which may be linked to Lyme disease. False positives or false negatives may occur prior to that time.

Fact

In 2005, according to the CDC, "23,305 cases of Lyme disease were reported, yielding a national average of 7.9 cases for every 100,000 persons. In the ten states where Lyme disease is most common, the average was 31.6 cases for every 100,000 persons."

Lyme disease is treated in its early stages with a two- to three-week course of oral antibiotics. If there are some other complications, intravenous antibiotics may be used. Antibiotics can be used if diagnosis is late or delayed, but there may be residual symptoms in such cases. Being treated early with antibiotics is your best chance for full recovery.

Prevention and Prevalence of Lyme Disease

Lyme was named in 1975 after an outbreak occurred in Lyme, Connecticut. It was discovered that people who work or spend leisure time in wooded areas, especially during tick season, were at higher risk of developing Lyme disease. To prevent the disease, make sure to wear protective clothing outdoors—long pants and long sleeves especially. It's also a good idea to use insect repellant with DEET, check for ticks when you come in from outside, clear away wooded, brushy, or grassy areas close to your home, and be aware of what the rash typical of Lyme disease looks like.

There is a peak of infection in the Northeast and Upper Midwest in late spring and early summer. A second peak period occurs in the fall. During late summer and winter, there is less chance of tick bites.

Raynaud's Phenomenon

Raynaud's phenomenon is a condition that affects blood vessels in the fingers, toes, ears, nose, and lips. During a Raynaud's attack the blood vessels constrict, which decreases blood flow. Typically, attacks last around fifteen minutes, but may last only one minute or up to several hours. When a Raynaud's attack occurs, there can be pain, numbness, tingling, swelling, throbbing, and discoloration of the affected digit or lobe. It is possible for sores to develop on the affected body part. Raynaud's attacks are often brought on by exposure to cold or periods of excessive stress.

Primary Raynaud's phenomenon is considered the more mild form of the condition. No other disease is associated with primary Raynaud's phenomenon. Secondary Raynaud's phenomenon is less common, yet more severe. Secondary Raynaud's phenomenon is associated with other connective-tissue diseases.

Diagnosing and Treating Raynaud's Phenomenon

Beyond a physical examination (which looks for blueness or pallor of the skin and redness with rewarming, as well as pitting scars or ulcers of the skin) and blood tests (sedrate and antinuclear antibody test) to rule out other rheumatic diseases, there are some specific diagnostic tests for Raynaud's phenomenon: nailfold capillaroscopy and a cold stimulation test.

Treatment of Raynaud's phenomenon is focused on preventing future attacks and permanent tissue damage. It is very important to warm the affected areas, keep yourself warm, manage your stress, stop smoking, relax, and exercise.

Medications such as calcium channel blockers, vasodilators, and smooth muscle relaxers are helpful. Surgery may be used in extreme cases. Usually, people adjust to living with Raynaud's phenomenon and are conscious of what can aggravate the condition.

Prevalence of Raynaud's Phenomenon

Approximately 85 to 95 percent of people with scleroderma or a mixed connective-tissue disease (MCTD) also have Raynaud's phenomenon. It is estimated that a third of lupus patients also have symptoms associated with Raynaud's phenomenon.

About 75 percent of all primary Raynaud's cases occur in women ages fifteen to forty. According to NIAMS, it has been estimated that Raynaud's phenomenon affects 5 to 10 percent of the general population in the United States, though estimates vary.

Alert

It is imperative for a person who suffers from Raynaud's phenomenon to keep warm. Wear gloves, even inside the house, if it helps. Rule number one is to protect yourself from the cold in any way you can.

Less Common Forms of Arthritis

There are many other types of arthritis and arthritis-related conditions that haven't yet been discussed. Here are ten more to consider:

Tendinitis—Tendons attach muscle to bone. Tendinitis is inflammation, swelling, or irritation of a tendon.

Bursitis—The bursa is a fluid-filled sac which lies between a tendon and skin, or between a tendon and bone. Bursitis is inflammation of the bursa sac.

Osteoporosis—Osteoporosis is a disease which causes bones to become less dense or brittle. Because of that, the bones are more prone to fracture. Several risk factors contribute to osteoporosis, including menopause and taking corticosteroids.

Costochondritis—Costochondritis is inflammation of a rib or the cartilage connecting a rib. It can cause chest pain that is indistinguishable from cardiac chest pain without an evaluation by a doctor.

Polymyositis—Polymyositis is a systemic connective-tissue disease characterized by inflammation and degeneration of the muscles. It is classified as a myopathy.

Dermatomyositis—Dermatomyositis is a connective-tissue disease that is characterized by inflammation of the muscles and the skin. Think of dermatomyositis as polymyositis plus skin inflammation. It is also classified as a myopathy.

Polymyalgia rheumatica—PMR is a rheumatic condition associated with moderate to severe muscle pain and stiffness in the neck, shoulder, and hip area.

Vasculitis—Vasculitis is inflammation of the blood vessels. Many rheumatic conditions are associated with vasculitis.

DISH—DISH is an acronym for Diffuse Idiopathic Skeletal Hyperostosis, which is a degenerative type of arthritis with calcification along the sides of the vertebrae.

Felty's syndrome—Felty's syndrome is a disorder characterized by rheumatoid arthritis, an enlarged spleen, a decreased white blood cell count, and recurrent infection.

Polyarthritis is one of the other common terms you may hear. Polyarthritis is any type of arthritis that affects five or more joints. Typically, polyarthritis implies one of the inflammatory types of arthritis.

CHAPTER 4

The Process of Diagnosing Arthritis

APPROPRIATE TREATMENT DEPENDS ON getting an accurate diagnosis. With so many different types of arthritis and symptoms that can overlap, diagnosis can be difficult in some cases. You may be inclined to try self-treatment initially, but as symptoms persist, a doctor must serve as the diagnostician. Determining which type of arthritis you have is a process. Your doctor will look for very specific signs, symptoms, and disease characteristics as the diagnosis is formulated. You should realize that the diagnostic process can take time, but it is worth it in order to get the most effective treatment.

Medical History

Your medical history is used to gather information about past medical conditions and your current medical condition. Details about symptoms you are currently experiencing and have experienced in the past are valuable to your doctor, who has the job of putting it all together. It's akin to assembling a jigsaw puzzle; with pieces of the puzzle in place, the picture becomes clearer. To obtain your medical history, you will likely be asked to fill out a questionnaire at your first appointment, and your doctor will ask you questions during each consultation.

Be Prepared for Questions

You will make the process easier for yourself and your doctor if you prepare ahead of time for some of the questions you will be asked. Having notes in hand can speed up the time it takes to fill out the written questionnaire. It's helpful for you to bring along:

- A list of medications and doses you are currently taking
- A list of medication allergies
- The names and contact information of other doctors you see, especially your primary doctor
- A list of prior surgeries
- Notes about medical conditions, past and present

During the consultation phase of your appointment, the questions your doctor asks will be based in part on the answers you provided on the written questionnaire. Your doctor will also ask more specific questions about symptoms. It is imperative that you give as much detail as possible and not conceal any symptoms you are experiencing. According to *U.S. News & World Report,* study results have shown that women with rheumatoid arthritis tend to downplay the severity of their symptoms when talking to doctors. Your doctor is likely to ask: how long you have had your current symptoms, if you have had a recent injury, if there is a pattern to when your symptoms occur or worsen, and how your symptoms limit your activities.

Stay on Topic

Most doctors are very busy. A good doctor tries to give ample time and attention to each individual patient, but you should realize that your doctor's time is valuable. You can help your doctor help you by staying on topic as you answer and ask questions. Don't hesitate to ask why something in your medical history is relevant, or inquire about anything you don't understand. Refrain from causing the conversation to drift; you have ground to cover and time is short.

Based on your answers, your doctor will formulate a preliminary diagnosis that may or may not be shared with you at this point. More information will be gathered from a physical examination and diagnostic tests.

Fact

According to the American College of Rheumatology, the average rheumatologist spends nearly fifty minutes with new patients and eighteen minutes with return patients. In an average week, the average rheumatologist in a single-specialty group sees eleven new patients and seventy-seven return patients.

Keep a Symptom Diary

At each subsequent visit to your doctor, you will be asked about your symptoms. You may be asked to rate your pain level on a 1-to-10 scale and about anything else your doctor should know, such as how you feel you are responding to prescribed treatments.

Doctor appointments may be closer together initially and spaced farther apart as a treatment plan is decided upon. It may become more difficult to recall symptom patterns or treatment side effects. To remember significant details, it may help you to keep a diary of symptoms or medical events. A diary may also help you and your doctor recognize patterns that are clinically significant.

Set up your diary to reflect the following: when you take your medications, how you feel each day or at specific times of day (include a pain scale), how you feel after taking medications or after any treatment, and how you feel after exercising or any other activity. It can also be helpful to include a description of sleep habits or patterns.

Your diary or journal will quickly become a daily habit. When you visit the doctor each time, you will have the information needed readily available. You will be able to relax and focus on what your doctor is telling you, rather than trying to remember what you need to tell your doctor.

Hands-On Physical Examination

A lot of information can be gathered from your medical history, but a hands-on physical examination performed by your doctor is also necessary to check on your current health status. During the physical examination, your doctor will be looking for visible symptoms, checking your range of motion, and observing changes in symptoms since your last physical examination.

Visible Symptoms

Your doctor will be looking for visible evidence during the physical examination. You will be observed for signs and symptoms that point to arthritis, including:

- Redness around the joint
- Warmth near the joint
- Joint stiffness
- Joint tenderness
- Fluid on a joint
- Bumps or nodules
- Pattern of affected joints
- Fever

As physical evidence is gathered, your doctor will work on a differential diagnosis, pitting one possible diagnosis against another. More diagnostic tests may be ordered before the working diagnosis is established. Treatment is prescribed based on the working diagnosis.

The criteria for diagnosis varies for the different types of arthritis. Classification criteria for rheumatic diseases appears on the American College of Rheumatology Web site at *www.rheumatology.org/publications/classification/index.asp.*

Range of Motion

During the physical examination, your doctor may check your range of motion to see how much deviation there is from the normal range of motion for a specific joint. Your doctor checks range of motion to assess limitation caused by existing joint damage or other symptoms such as joint swelling, muscle spasms, and pain associated with arthritis. It is also helpful to establish a baseline measurement so future improvement or decline in range of motion can be tracked.

Range of motion is measured using a goniometer. Several types of goniometers exist, but the most common is a 180-degree, double-armed goniometer. As your doctor checks your range of motion, the joint movements that will be observed include: flexion (bending), extension (straightening), abduction (moving out or away from midline of the body), and rotation.

Range of motion, if impaired, reduces the distance and direction you can move your joint. As arthritis limits range of motion, mobility and function can be affected. Preserving range of motion is one of the goals of arthritis treatment.

Observing Change in Symptoms

It is important to recognize and report any increase or decrease in the severity of arthritis symptoms. It's also important to let your doctor know about any new symptoms you have developed. Symptoms reflect disease activity and the effectiveness or ineffectiveness of your current treatment.

Question

What is the difference between active and passive range of motion?
Moving your own joint through its range of motion is referred to as active range of motion. If your doctor moves your joint through its range of motion, that is referred to as passive range of motion.

Since arthritis symptoms vary from patient to patient, your doctor will be monitoring your individual progress. If you think of symptoms as indicators, it will help you convey changes in symptoms to your doctor. Your specific indicators will help you and your doctor make decisions about your treatment plan.

It's also useful to convey what you may have done to cause a change in symptoms. Try to answer these questions:

- What activity caused your joint to swell?
- What did you do to relieve the swelling?
- What activity may have caused your joint to stiffen?
- What, if anything, relieved the stiffness?
- What caused your pain level to increase?
- What relieves your pain and makes it tolerable?
- Is the stiffness worse in the morning?
- How long does it take to achieve maximum improvement?
- Do your symptoms get worse or better with activity?

Don't forget, it's just as important to disclose symptoms that have improved as symptoms that have worsened. Symptoms that have improved confirm that your treatment plan is working; the opposite can be said of worsening symptoms. The observations of doctor and patient are both relevant and form the foundation for making future decisions about your treatment goals.

Blood Tests

After a medical history is given and a physical examination is performed, your doctor may still need more information. Laboratory tests, especially blood tests, can provide a lot of information beyond what the medical history or physical examination can provide. You should ask your doctor about the tests being ordered. It will help you understand the diagnostic process and know what your doctor is looking for, rather than feeling unsure about the orders you have in hand. By ordering blood tests, your doctor is able to not only confirm a diagnosis, but monitor disease activity and the effectiveness of your medications or treatments. Through blood tests he can also be alerted to any side effects possibly caused by your medications

There are blood tests that you should expect your doctor to order when you are first being evaluated and some which will continue to be ordered routinely. Laboratory tests are important but not perfect diagnostic tools.

Alert

There can be false positive or false negative blood-test results. You may have arthritis, but tests may not reveal it, especially at first. On the contrary, you may have a blood test result suggestive of arthritis but never have the disease.

Rheumatoid Factor

Rheumatoid factor (RF) is an antibody or immunoglobulin present in about 70 to 80 percent of adults who have rheumatoid arthritis. Some people with other chronic inflammatory conditions, and up to 5 percent of healthy individuals, are also positive for rheumatoid factor.

The test for rheumatoid factor is performed using latex agglutination or nephelometry. If your test result is positive for rheumatoid factor, your blood sample is further analyzed using serial dilutions to obtain a *titer* (serial dilutions of the patient's blood still yielding a positive result). Using the latex agglutination test, a titer greater than 1:20 is abnormal. High titers also correlate with severity of the disease. For example, 1:320 is likely to reflect a more severe course of rheumatoid arthritis than 1:40. Using nephelometry, a result of more than 23 units and a titer more than 1:80 is abnormal. Some rheumatoid factor tests are now reported in IU (international units).

Essential

A negative result for the rheumatoid factor test does not exclude the possibility of having rheumatoid arthritis. About 20 percent of people with rheumatoid arthritis are negative for rheumatoid factor and classified as having seronegative rheumatoid arthritis.

Erythrocyte Sedimentation Rate

The erythrocyte sedimentation rate (ESR) is commonly referred to as sedimentation rate or sedrate. The test is an indicator of the presence of nonspecific inflammation. The patient's blood sample is placed in a special graduated tube and allowed to sit undisturbed for an hour. Red cells fall at a faster rate if inflammation is present.

The normal value for sedrate is less than or equal to 10mm/hour for men and less than or equal to 20 mm/hour for women. Normal ranges do increase with age. Though the test is not specific regarding the origin of the inflammation, it is used as an indicator of severity of inflammation.

C-Reactive Protein (CRP)

C-reactive protein is a protein produced by the liver following tissue injury. Plasma levels of CRP increase quickly following periods of acute inflammation or infection, making this test a better indicator of disease activity than the sedrate, which changes more gradually. In chronic diseases, the test is used to monitor the effectiveness of treatments. The normal level of CRP is less than 1.0 mg/dl.

Anti-Cyclic Citrullinated Peptide Antibody Test (Anti-CCP)

The anti-cyclic citrullinated peptide antibody anti-CCP that become more common. The test is ordered if rheumatoid arthritis is suspected. Moderate to high levels of anti-CCP in a patient's blood confirm the diagnosis of rheumatoid arthritis. The test is more specific than rheumatoid factor, which can be positive even though a person doesn't have rheumatoid arthritis. Higher levels of anti-CCP also predict a more severe course of rheumatoid arthritis.

Antinuclear Antibodies (ANA)

Antinuclear antibodies (ANA) are abnormal autoantibodies (immunoglobulins against nuclear components of the human cell). The test is sometimes referred to as FANA or fluorescent antinuclear antibody test since it is based on indirect immunofluorescence.

Moderate to high antinuclear antibody levels are suggestive of autoimmune disease. Low levels are seen in about 5 percent of healthy adults. Positive antinuclear antibody tests are seen in:

- More than 95 percent of systemic lupus erythematosus patients
- 60 to 80 percent of systemic sclerosis (scleroderma) patients
- 40 to 70 percent of patients with Sjögren's syndrome
- 30 to 80 percent of patients with polymyositis or dermatomyositis
- 20 to 60 percent of patients with Raynaud's phenomenon
- 30 to 50 percent of rheumatoid arthritis patients
- 5 to 25 percent of patients with discoid lupus

Positive ANA test results are reported in titers and patterns. Common patterns include homogeneous, speckled, nucleolar, centromere, and cytoplasmic. The pattern, which is viewed on specially prepared slides under a fluorescent microscope, has become less significant since more specific autoantibody tests have been developed.

Antinuclear antibodies can be negative during remissions or periods of low disease activity. Since ANA titers are increased during flares, the ANA test can reflect disease activity and help formulate disease prognosis. However, if the ANA is positive, it typically is always positive, so it may not be the best blood test to follow disease activity.

Complete Blood Count and Platelet Count

The complete blood count determines the WBC (white blood-cell count), RBC (red blood-cell count), hemoglobin, hematocrit, and several red blood-cell indices. Elevated white blood-cell counts suggest the possibility of an active infection. Patients taking corticosteroids may have an elevated WBC due to the medication. Chronic inflammation can cause a low red blood-cell count. Low hemoglobin and hematocrit may be indicative of anemia associated with chronic diseases or possible bleeding caused by medications. The platelet count is often high in rheumatoid arthritis patients, while some potent arthritis medications can cause platelets to be low.

📋 Fact

It is possible for a rheumatoid arthritis patient to have a normal CRP and sedrate. In rare cases, there appears to be low sensitivity or inability to trigger the liver to produce inflammatory proteins required for both tests.

HLA Tissue Typing

Human leukocyte antigens (HLA) are proteins on the surface of cells. Specific HLA proteins are genetic markers for some of the rheumatic diseases. Patients may be tested to see if they have the genetic markers. HLA-B27 has been associated with ankylosing spondylitis and other spondyloarthropathies. Rheumatoid arthritis is associated with HLA-DR4.

Uric Acid

Elevated levels of uric acid in the blood (known as hyperuricemia) can cause crystals to form, which are deposited in the joints and tissues, causing painful gout attacks. Uric acid is the final product of purine metabolism in humans. Not everyone who has elevated uric acid will develop gout. A blood uric-acid level greater than 7 for men and greater than 6 for women is considered elevated. Elevated uric acid can result from excess production in the body or insufficient elimination.

Radiographic Studies (X-Rays)

X-rays are the oldest and most commonly used type of medical imaging. Your doctor may order x-rays (radiographs), which are essentially pictures of your bones and joints. X-rays don't show cartilage, muscles, or ligaments. X-rays use electromagnetic radiation and are considered a very safe form of medical imaging. An x-ray machine is used to focus an x-ray beam on a specific part of the body to capture the images on x-ray film or record the images digitally.

Reading X-Rays

Bone and metal show up white on an x-ray because they are dense and block the x-ray beam, decreasing exposure of the film to the x-ray beam. Shades of gray on the x-ray represent soft tissue of various sizes and densities. Air appears black on x-ray.

Your doctor will be looking for evidence of joint damage or bone abnormalities on the x-ray images. It's possible to have evidence of abnormalities that are associated with aging, irrespective of pain or other symptoms. It's also possible to have normal x-rays even though you have inflammation, which is symptomatic.

A person is generally exposed to about 20 milliroentgens of radiation during a single x-ray exposure. The amount of radiation will be based on the body part to be x-rayed (e.g., a pelvic x-ray has much more radiation than a chest x-ray). To put it in perspective, each year every person is exposed to about 100 milliroentgens of radiation from sources like the sun and soil.

Question

Are x-rays safe for arthritis patients?
Some patients worry about the safety of x-rays. Some fear the exposure to radiation may eventually cause cancer. The cumulative effect of x-rays is also a concern; however, there is no scientific data indicating danger associated with diagnostic x-rays.

Magnetic Resonance Imaging (MRI)

MRI scans produce cross-sectional images of your body by using a magnetic field, radio waves, and a computer. Information about bones, joints, and soft tissues is provided with precision.

An MRI machine or scanner is actually a tube surrounded by a large circular magnet. The magnetic field is created by passing electric current through coils contained in the housing of the machine for the purpose of aligning the protons of the body. Other coils emit radio waves that spin the protons and produce a faint signal. The signals are collected by the computer to produce an image. Very small changes in the body can be detected using MRI. If an MRI is ordered for you remember to: Tell the technician if you have metal implants or electronic medical devices in your body; tell the technician if you are claustrophobic; and remove any jewelry or metal accessories prior to the test.

An MRI scan is a painless procedure. The only discomfort may come from lying in one position during the test or the clanking noises produced by the MRI machine. Earphones are provided to reduce the noise. An MRI can take from thirty to ninety minutes. If you can remain calm and relaxed, it will go smoothly. You must lie still because any movement will blur the images.

Some doctors order contrast with the MRI scan. You may have an IV started at the beginning of your scan and at some point during the MRI scan a contrast agent is injected into the IV site. The purpose of the contrast is to obtain a better view of certain tissues.

Fact

There is contradictory information circulating about whether or not a patient who has a joint replacement can have an MRI scan. The magnetic field and metal implant may cause a problem; however, it depends on what type of metal is in the implant. Your doctor has that information and should be contacted prior to scheduling an MRI.

Your rheumatologist may order an MRI of your hand to establish a baseline for rheumatoid arthritis patients. Subsequent MRIs of the hand detect changes that correlate with disease progression. If there are no significant changes, that would suggest disease progression may have slowed and your treatment plan is effective.

Joint Aspiration

Useful diagnostic information can be obtained from synovial fluid (joint fluid) removed from a joint using a needle and syringe. The procedure, called a joint aspiration, can be performed in a doctor's office. The procedure is also referred to as synovial fluid analysis, joint tap, or arthrocentesis and is used to find out what is causing joint pain or joint swelling.

The Procedure

Removing or draining the joint fluid may actually have a side benefit of relieving any pressure or pain it is causing at the joint. A joint aspiration can be performed at the same time as a joint injection.

Joint aspiration and injection is easier, and therefore more common, in some joints. Knees are easy to aspirate and inject. Shoulders, elbows, wrists, thumbs, small joints of the hands and feet, and ankles may also be aspirated and injected. Hip joints, which are less easy to access, may need to be done via a guided procedure using x-ray or ultrasound for that purpose.

Specimen Analysis

The joint fluid specimen is examined microscopically for bacteria, crystals, and blood cells. Sometimes levels of glucose, protein, and LDH (lactic dehydrogenase) are measured. The color and clarity of the joint fluid is also observed and reported.

Parameters found on a normal joint-fluid report include a clear to light yellow appearance, no or few blood cells, no crystals present, and no bacteria seen microscopically or grown in culture. In a normal report, protein will be less than 3 g/dl, glucose will be greater than or equal to 40 mg/dl, and there will be an LDH level of 105–333 IU/L.

Abnormal joint-fluid results have a cloudy (indicative of infection or inflammation)—or bloody (indicative of bleeding) appearance.

Abnormal results also have large numbers of blood cells (red blood cells would suggest bleeding in the joint while white blood cells suggest gout, pseudogout, inflammatory forms of arthritis, injury, or infection). A large number of white cells would go against injury, while a large number of red cells would favor an injury. Crystals will also be present (uric-acid crystals are indicative of gout; calcium pyrophosphate dihydrate crystals are indicative of pseudogout) and bacteria will be seen microscopically or grown in culture (indicative of infection). A protein level of greater than or equal to 3 g/dl (which suggests inflammation or infection) represents abnormal results, as does a glucose level of less than 40 mg/dl (suggests inflammation or infection). The LDH level will be greater than 333 IU/L (rheumatoid arthritis, gout, or infection are suspected with high LDH in joint fluid, but normal LDH level in blood).

Differential white blood-cell counts can be done on joint fluid. The predominance of certain types of white cells can help distinguish a septic joint or an inflammatory type of arthritis from a crystal-induced arthropathy.

Other Diagnostic Tests

There are other less commonly ordered tests that may be necessary for some patients. These are usually ordered to confirm a diagnosis or check for adverse effects of treatment.

Blood Profiles and Urine Tests

Kidney profiles and liver profiles (blood tests) are sometimes ordered to check that medications you may be taking are not damaging or impairing the normal function of those organs.

Blood tests that are done to test for kidney damage include BUN or blood urea nitrogen (normal is 7–20 mg/dl) and serum creatinine (normal is 0.8–1.2 mg/dl for males and 0.6–0.9 mg/dl for females).

Urine tests are also used to check for kidney damage. These tests include urinalysis (includes many parameters), urea clearance (normal is 64–99 ml/min), and creatinine clearance (normal for adults under forty years old is 90–139 ml/min for males and 80–125 ml/min for females). For adults over forty years old, the normal decreases 6.5ml/min for each decade. There is also the urine osmolality (normal is 50–1400 mOsm/kg for random specimen) and a 24-hour urine protein test (normal is less than or equal to 150 mg of protein).

Liver enzymes are also analyzed to check for side effects of arthritis medications. These include AST (SGOT) with a normal range of 10–34 IU/L (international units per liter), ALT (SGPT) with a normal range of 5–35 IU/L, ALP with a normal range of 20–140 IU/L, and GGT or GGTP with a normal range of 0–51 IU/L.

Bilirubin, albumin, total protein, and prothrombin time are also tests helpful in determining liver function.

Biopsies

Biopsies are ordered to confirm a diagnosis or assess disease activity. A biopsy involves the removal of a small piece of tissue that is then prepared for microscopic examination. Biopsies of the skin, muscle, and kidney are the most commonly performed biopsies for arthritis patients.

For arthritis patients, skin biopsies are used to diagnose lupus, vasculitis, psoriatic arthritis, or other types of arthritis that have skin involvement. Muscle biopsies are used to diagnose polymyositis or vasculitis. Kidney biopsies help diagnose lupus. Liver biopsies are used to check for damage in patients taking methotrexate. Biopsy of minor salivary glands in the mouth is helpful in confirming a diagnosis of Sjögren's syndrome, and biopsy of the synovial lining of a joint helps rule out an indolent infection such as tuberculosis or fungus.

Other Imaging Techniques

There are more highly specialized imaging techniques available, such as arthrography, which involves injecting dye into your joint so more details are visible on the x-ray.

An isotope bone scan involves a small amount of radioactive isotope injected into your blood. The isotope is taken up by your bones and gives off gamma rays. After a special camera detects the gamma rays, a computer receives the information and builds an image that shows where bones are inflamed.

CT scans use x-rays which record images of sections of the body. A computer creates cross-sectional pictures from the information. Detailed pictures of the skeleton as well as muscles and other tissues are created. CT scans transmit a much larger amount of radiation than plain radiographs.

DEXA (dual energy x-ray absorptiometry) scans are used to evaluate bone density and are primarily used to diagnose osteoporosis, a condition of bone thinning. Radiation is minimal for DEXA scans.

Ultrasound uses high frequency sound waves to create pictures. It is useful for locating the abnormal presence of fluid around joints and tendons.

CHAPTER 5

Your Doctor Works for You

WITH SYMPTOMS THAT SEEM TO HAVE appeared out of nowhere and without cause, you probably feel confused about what to do. Whether your arthritis symptoms came on gradually or suddenly, if symptoms persist, consulting your doctor is the right action to take. Your primary care doctor will make a preliminary determination to decide if referring you to a rheumatologist or orthopedic specialist is necessary. Depending on the range of your symptoms, you may require a team of doctors and health-care professionals. Remember that you are on the team, not just a spectator. Your doctors work for you and serve as your advisors.

Should You See a Rheumatologist?

A board-certified rheumatologist is a medical doctor (an internal medicine doctor or pediatrician) who specializes in the diagnosis and treatment of arthritis and other rheumatic diseases. Rheumatologists have an extensive background that includes four years of medical school, three years of training in internal medicine or pediatrics, plus two or three more years training in rheumatology. To become a board-certified rheumatologist, doctors must pass an extensive exam at the end of their training.

Clearly, rheumatologists have the most experience with diagnosing and treating arthritic conditions. Some rheumatologists focus on research while others focus on patient care. Some devote time to both research and patient care. There are obvious benefits to having a doctor who is on the cutting edge of arthritis news and research.

The complexity of your initial symptoms is a deciding factor in whether you need a rheumatologist. Internal medicine doctors and orthopedists also treat arthritis patients. Some patients may see a rheumatologist just to ensure an accurate diagnosis and decide on a course of treatment. After that, they may follow up with their primary care doctor or an orthopedist. Other patients consult with their rheumatologist on a regular basis. Factors such as your insurance requirements and your location may dictate how often you see a rheumatologist; access to a rheumatologist can be difficult for some people to achieve.

 Alert

According to the American College of Rheumatology, there is a shortage of rheumatologists. Some areas, especially rural ones, have no rheumatologists within close proximity. The problem, which is expected to worsen without more funding earmarked for education and training, is burdensome to arthritis patients as well as current rheumatologists.

If you haven't been referred to a rheumatologist but feel you should see a specialist, discuss it with your primary care doctor. You can request a referral or make an appointment on your own. If you are undecided about whether you should consult with a rheumatologist, review this checklist to help you decide.

- Do you have persistent joint pain and swelling that has lasted longer than two weeks and may be arthritis?
- Do you have tenderness that becomes worse with movement or activity?
- Do you have joints that are red and warm, possibly indicative of inflammation?
- Have you lost range of motion in the affected joint or joints?

- Have you experienced unexplained weight loss?
- Do you have a fever, extreme fatigue, or a general feeling of being not well?
- Have your symptoms interfered with your work or usual daily activities?
- Are you uncertain of your diagnosis?

If you answered yes to any of the questions on the checklist, you should consult with a rheumatologist.

Rheumatology is one of the lowest paid of all internal-medicine subspecialties, and there are too few newly graduated doctors choosing to specialize in rheumatology. At the same time, there are many practicing rheumatologists nearing retirement. Coupled with the fact that the population is aging and the baby-boomer generation is developing arthritis, a crisis in the rheumatology specialty is developing. The shortage may make it more difficult for you to find a rheumatologist near you or you may have to wait longer than expected for an appointment.

To find a well-respected, highly recommended rheumatologist, your first resource should be a referral from your primary doctor. You may be offered more than one choice or wish to find your own rheumatologist.

The American College of Rheumatology offers a geographical directory of rheumatologists on its Web site at *www.rheumatology .org/directory/geo.asp?aud=pat*. You can search rheumatologists by name or location in the United States and other countries.

Your local office of the Arthritis Foundation can be found at this Web site, *www.arthritis.org/communities/Chapters/ChapDirectory .asp*, and can provide you with names of rheumatologists.

Neither the American College of Rheumatology nor the Arthritis Foundation make recommendations, however. The Internet may be of help in finding non-biased Web sites that have accumulated information about top doctors in your area. An example might include *www.bestdoctors.com*.

What You Should Expect During Office Visits

Before you see your rheumatologist, a nurse or medical assistant will likely weigh you and check your vital signs. You will be asked about your chief complaints with regard to recent symptoms. Then the nurse or medical assistant will leave your chart outside the room while you wait for your doctor.

With your rheumatologist, you can expect to discuss the results of any tests you may have had since your last appointment. Abnormal results should be explained to you and you should also be informed about which parameters are within normal limits. Your rheumatologist will then turn his attention to your current complaints. This is your time to communicate any problems, issues, or concerns that you have to your rheumatologist. He will summarize your conversation in your medical record so there will be continuity with future appointments.

He will then ask you specific questions about your pain level and pain patterns, and will also look for swelling, redness, and warmth around your joints. You will be observed for joint tenderness, nodules, joint deformity, and rashes, and your range of motion will be tested. You may have more diagnostic tests ordered to check on systemic effects.

L. Essential

> Be prepared to jot down important details or new medical terms, but at the same time be brief with note taking so it isn't distracting to your doctor. Be attentive while your doctor is speaking; you don't want to be the patient who leaves the doctor's office and says, "I don't remember what was just said."

The information gathered from your conversation and physical examination give your rheumatologist a snapshot of how you have improved or declined since your last appointment. If new problems have developed, your rheumatologist will decide on an appropriate treatment plan or an adjustment to your current treatment plan.

You may be referred to another specialist if further assessment is indicated.

Your rheumatologist not only assesses your physical status; the impact of your disease on mental, social, and work aspects, and daily living will also be discussed. Your rheumatologist can help you with many areas of your life that are impacted by your disease. Approach him with anything that is concerning you related to your medical condition. He is much more than a prescription pad.

Consider anything you may need from your rheumatologist such as a referral to physical therapy, a surgical consult with an orthopedic surgeon, or a letter to support your application for disability. You may also want your rheumatologist to talk to your family and explain your situation or discuss what you might need in order to take a leave of absence from work.

Your rheumatologist is not a wizard. He can't make a bad marriage good again or make your disease disappear. There are many ways your rheumatologist can realistically help you, though.

Rheumatologists are pivotal people in the lives of their patients. Ideally, you want to be able to say, "My rheumatologist is like a member of my family," or "I feel so much better after I leave my rheumatologist's office. I feel like I have been heard and that he gets it."

Results from a telephone survey of 192 patients, published in the Mayo Clinic Proceedings in 2006, revealed how they felt doctors should appear:

- Confident
- Empathetic
- Forthright
- Humane
- Personal
- Respectful
- Thorough

Patients do not want their doctor to be:

- Timid
- Uncaring
- Misleading
- Cold
- Callous
- Disrespectful
- Hurried

Compare your doctor to the traits listed. Does your doctor have more ideal traits or more traits that are not ideal? If your doctor has shortcomings, do you consider them bothersome or minor annoyances? Remember, since you have a chronic disease, your doctor will play a significant role in your life.

Questions Ready and Welcomed?

During your initial appointment and at all subsequent appointments, you must attempt to understand what you're told about your diagnosis and treatment plan. Compliance with your treatment plan in large part depends on understanding the reasons behind decisions being made.

It's your responsibility to follow along, and to do that you will need to ask a lot of questions, so it's important to have a doctor who is open to questions. An excellent doctor is one who is knowledgeable, keeps current with new developments in his specialty, and realizes that patient comprehension is half of the battle.

Here are twenty-one questions to ask your doctor. Use it as a guide for developing more of your own questions. If you don't know an answer to any of the following questions, the question needs to be asked.

- Have you confirmed that I have arthritis?
- What type of arthritis do I have?
- What treatment plan are you recommending?
- How should I take my medications (e.g., with or without food)?
- What is the mechanism of action for each medication?
- Are you prescribing the brand name or generic version of the drugs?
- What are the possible side effects associated with each medication?
- If I experience side effects, what should I do?

- When should I expect to notice any improvement in my condition?
- How long should I stay on a medication if I'm not noticing any improvement?
- What options should I know about if I decide I need to switch medications?
- Will I need routine blood tests to monitor progress and side effects?
- When and how will I be able to get results of any tests that have been done?
- What complementary treatments do you recommend along with my medications?
- Am I able to speak directly with you on the phone if I need to call with questions?
- Under what conditions should I go directly to the emergency room?
- With which hospitals are you affiliated?
- What is the usual prognosis for my condition?
- Will I ever be able to stop taking all medications?
- How often will I need to come back to consult with you?
- Do I need to stop or modify any of my usual activities?

Your doctor's willingness to answer all of your questions is a sign of good communication. The more you see your doctor, you might expect there to be fewer general questions and more specific questions. Write down your questions as you think of them. Having a prepared list will help both you and your doctor focus on the task at hand, which is helping you.

If your doctor discourages questions, that can be reason enough to find a new doctor. Just as with any relationship, you and your doctor need to become familiar with what you each expect and how you both do things. As long as your questions get answered, do you care if your doctor prefers you ask them only at the end of the appointment? Does your doctor mind that you arrive with notes, or does she expect that you will and even encourage it? You and your doctor need to create ground rules that are agreeable to you both. Work toward developing an effective doctor-patient relationship that you will depend on for years to come.

Should You Understand Everything Your Doctor Says?

The short answer is yes, as much as possible. The more you understand about your condition and what to expect going forward, the less anxious you will feel. Patients who feel they understand feel they are in control of their disease.

If you find comfort in bringing along a family member or friend, do it. Keep your group small because the focus needs to remain on you. Your family and friends can provide more ears with which to listen, learn, and understand.

Health Literacy

Your doctor may at times use medical terms you don't understand. Never hesitate to ask what something means and don't just let it go. Learning is vitally important to achieving your treatment goals.

Fact

According to the Institute of Medicine, health literacy is defined as the degree to which a person has the capacity to obtain, process, and understand basic information and services needed to make appropriate decisions about their health. About 90 million people, or half of all American adults, have a problem with understanding and using health information.

Limited health literacy leads to a higher rate of hospitalization and emergency room use, as well as billions of dollars spent on avoidable health-care costs. Getting back to you specifically, could you feel comfortable not knowing what's wrong, why a test is being ordered, or why a treatment plan is being recommended over another? You need clarity as much as you need your treatment.

Use reputable sources to learn about health information. The Internet makes health information easily accessible. Choose a few great Web sites you can trust and stick with them. You will feel comfortable formulating questions for your doctor if you feel you have first developed a base of knowledge yourself.

Can You Know Too Much?

Patient education promotes better understanding. The emphasis is on understanding. Patient education is not for the purpose of empowering you improperly. Examples of improper empowerment are if you feel you are smarter than your doctor, you feel you can make your health decisions without your doctor's advice, you only need your doctor to write prescriptions for you, and patient education has diminished the trust and respect you had for your doctor.

Patient education should enhance the doctor-patient relationship by allowing you to comprehend and communicate intelligently with your doctor. If you feel improperly empowered or if your doctor feels threatened by your approach, you both may need to reassess your roles.

Ask your doctor to recommend resources where you can learn more about your disease and treatment options. Even as you become more informed, never will you reach the point where your doctor's advice isn't valuable. Your best chance to do all you can do to improve your health and cope with your disease comes with your doctor as team leader and you on the team as well. The greatest doctor-patient relationships have these roles clearly defined.

If you are uneasy about asking questions when you're with your doctor, discuss it and get your doctor's feelings regarding informed versus uninformed patients. Ask when it is the best time to ask questions. Work with your doctor to develop a routine that works for you— a routine that allows for questions and explanations. Your doctor will appreciate that you were open about your need to understand.

How to Tell if It's Time to Change Doctors

Continuity of care is important. Following through with a doctor's assessment and treatment recommendations makes sense, unless there are problems and issues that interfere. There are reasons that may necessitate moving on to another doctor. Some patients, though not satisfied with their doctor, maintain the relationship because they just don't know how to move on. How do you tell a doctor you're not coming back? How do you find a new doctor more suitable to your needs? If you find yourself in that situation, make your needs the priority. A positive relationship with your doctor boosts your effort to improve your health and live well with arthritis.

Not every patient appreciates the same type of doctor. Some doctors explain medical information in detail while others are brief with explanations. Some doctors are better listeners than others.

Essential

A doctor's personality is not reflective of their ability to diagnose and treat patients, but it may make a difference in your responsiveness. You need to feel comfortable with your doctor. Consider how you feel when you leave your doctor's office. That's a good indication of your overall satisfaction.

Trust and Confidence

The foundation for a lasting doctor-patient relationship is trust. You must trust in your doctor's ability. You must trust in your doctor's advice, guidance, and judgment and feel that you're being told everything you need to know. If you have trust, feelings of apprehension disappear. If you lack trust, your confidence in the whole process will erode.

Communication

The issue of communication is two-fold. For you to be compliant with your treatment plan, you need to be fully informed regarding why certain decisions are being made; most people don't comply with what they don't understand. You need a doctor who is forthcoming with information pertinent to your condition. You must feel assured that your doctor believes the time spent helping you understand is time well spent.

After your doctor offers a thorough explanation of what you need to know, you should be encouraged to ask questions and clarify anything that is still not completely clear.

Conversations between you and your doctor should not feel strained, tense, or awkward, even when the discussion gets complicated. Your conversations should help you decompress, not stress.

Continuity Between Visits

Your doctor is a busy person and sees many patients every day. When it's your turn in the office, your doctor should be up to speed on your medical file, and be able to recall exactly where you left off during your previous visit. There is something unsettling about a doctor who has to fumble through the pages of your medical record in search of a starting point. If you sense your doctor is lost, your intuition is probably correct. Everyone has a bad day now and again, but just as time is valuable to your doctor, time is valuable to you as well.

You may not have an optimal situation if you need to remind your doctor what tests were ordered last visit, your doctor repeatedly can't find test results in your file, if you had a bad test result but were not called and informed, and if you have to remind your doctor that it's time to have a routine or repeat test. It's common sense that continuity of care will work in your favor, and you should not settle for less.

Inconveniences

There are more practical problems that might make a doctor unsuitable for you. Certainly, you must check that your doctor is available to you through your health-insurance plan. Many plans have preferred provider lists and you will need to choose your doctor from the list or consider that there may be an extra expense to see a physician who is not on your provider list. Other considerations include:

Location—Determine how far away from your residence you are willing to drive to your appointments. If possible, the location should not be a burden for you.

Reaching your doctor—If an unforeseen problem develops, how accessible is your doctor to you? Can you talk to him directly on the telephone? Can a nurse get a message to your doctor quickly and call you back? Is there an answering service taking messages after hours?

Short notice—If you need an appointment before the one you already have scheduled, how difficult is it to get in to see your doctor? Is it possible to be added on at the end of the day or first thing in the morning?

Long waiting lists—If you are a referral patient, is the wait to get an appointment unreasonable? Are you being offered an appointment many weeks or even months away and longer than you feel you can wait?

These are issues that matter to patients in varying degrees. You can see, though, that the more things you feel are right and the fewer things that seem wrong will work in your favor.

Before you decide to switch doctors, consider getting a second opinion. It will put you at ease if the second opinion concurs with the recommendations of your regular doctor and it gives you the opportunity to compare the two doctors.

If you still feel you need to change doctors, you have the option of not explaining why you won't be returning. Contact the office personnel for a copy of your medical records. You also have the option of discussing the issues with your doctor, giving it one last chance to see if it's a workable situation. If not and you still decide to move on, informing your doctor of your reasons may actually help the doctor improve on weaknesses.

Coordinating Your Doctors

If you have several doctors treating several different conditions, one doctor needs to take on the role of coordinator of your health care. Comorbid conditions may present overlapping symptoms; to prevent confusion and duplication, your medical records and test results should be made available to every doctor who is caring for you so they are all sharing the same pertinent facts.

Your Responsibility in Coordinating Your Doctors

Be sure all of your doctors are on the same page. Ask Doctor A's office if Doctors B, C, and D are getting copies of your reports and test results. Follow up when you see the other doctors to make sure they received the reports they should have received—don't just assume they did. Your medical care should be a coordinated and unified effort. Though your rheumatologist or primary care doctor will serve the role of coordinator, some of the responsibility is still yours.

Second Opinions

Some patients will see a doctor other than their regular doctor for a second opinion. The doctor who is expected to offer a second opinion has little to no history on you. The doctor will base his opinion on the information you provide and whatever tests the doctor wants repeated or ordered for the first time.

Since the second-opinion doctors usually only see the patient for one or a few consultations, some have speculated that second opinions don't always add up. Dr. Scott Haig, a columnist for Time.com, suggested that marketing has shaped medicine into a patient-driven system, often inefficient and expensive. Haig rhetorically asks if compensating a good doctor properly wouldn't create a more efficient kind of health care, instead of patients being passed from one doctor to another.

There are some sound reasons for getting a second opinion, however. You may want to learn if another doctor agrees with your diagnosis or can offer different treatment options. Your doctor may recommend that you seek a second opinion and your health-insurance plan may even require it before approving a specific procedure.

The Problem with Having Multiple Doctors

With multiple doctors writing multiple prescriptions, you need to be sure of what was prescribed. Check that you can read the prescription before you leave your doctor's office. Have your doctor repeat the name of the medication and review the instructions; it's important for you to follow along. Consider how many patients a doctor sees each week and how many prescriptions he writes: Doctors are human and the potential for mistakes exists. With your help, mistakes can be prevented, including: duplicate prescriptions for the same drug, prescriptions for a combination of drugs that can interact and cause adverse reaction, errors on the written prescription, and duplication of diagnostic tests

Some patients are comfortable leaving it all up to the doctors. Doctors are professionals, so it seems counterintuitive that the patient would have to double check anything. Think back about four decades; in the 1960s, doctors were actually revered by their patients.

CHAPTER 6

Treating Arthritis

WHILE RESEARCHERS WORK TOWARD finding a cure for arthritis, arthritis symptoms can be managed with an effective treatment plan. Newly diagnosed patients quickly learn that arthritis treatment is not one-size-fits-all; it is a process, and sometimes a long one, to determine the best course of treatment.

It's not unusual for established patients who have been treated for many years to change their course of treatment for various reasons. Whether a patient is new or established, the goal of treatment is to minimize symptoms, prevent joint damage, slow disease progression, and maintain joint function and mobility.

Self-Treatment

You may, like many others, decide to self-treat when you first experience symptoms. With the hope that the problem is minor and will go away, you may try self-treating with over-the-counter pain relievers or using even more conservative treatment (e.g., heat, ice, rest, supplements). There is a place for self-treatment in arthritis management, but not without evaluation by a medical professional.

With over 100 types of arthritis, each having different treatment options, it's necessary for you to be diagnosed accurately first. Think of your diagnosis as a cogwheel that sets everything in motion, so you can develop a strategy with your doctor for treatment and management of the disease.

The principle taught to all medical students seems to also apply to patients with regard to self-treatment: First do no harm. You must act cautiously. If you feel inclined to try over-the-counter anti-inflammatory medications and pain medications, dietary and herbal supplements, or any one of myriad concoctions that claim to cure arthritis, you should consult your doctor about everything you intend to try. You should not begin to self-treat without the knowledge of potential side effects, adverse reactions, or possible drug interactions.

Essential

The Arthritis Foundation recommends seeing a doctor if you have joint pain, stiffness, or swelling which persists for two or more weeks, whether or not your symptoms began suddenly or gradually. Arthritis can only be diagnosed by a doctor, and proper treatment depends on a proper diagnosis.

For example, acetaminophen or Tylenol can cause liver damage or death if the maximum allowable daily dose (4000 mg or 8 extra-strength caplets) is exceeded. The cumulative amount of acetaminophen in multiple OTC products must also be considered.

For joint health, there is glucosamine, MSM, and SAMe sold as dietary supplements. Acetaminophen is a pain reliever sold over-the-counter. Ibuprofen, Naprosyn, and Ketoprofen are nonsteroidal anti-inflammatory medications also sold over-the-counter in a strength which is less than prescription strength. Topical creams are also popular self-treatments for arthritis.

If you do actually have one of the more severe types of arthritis, the time spent pursuing useless or ineffective treatments takes valuable time away from starting early, aggressive treatment, which is the current recommendation.

Certain aspects of self-treatment are definitely good for you and may be incorporated into your treatment plan after you have been diagnosed. Tips for healthy self-treatment include:

- Follow joint protection principles
- Balance activity and rest
- Use relaxation techniques
- Maintain a healthy weight
- Stop smoking

Your self-care regimen should still be documented in your medical record at your doctor's office. Studies have shown that patients who work with their doctor to develop their treatment plan are more likely to be compliant and feel better about their care. Together with your doctor, you will decide which aspects of prescribed care and self-care should be used together, with the goal being to improve your health.

℞ Alert

Over-the-counter (OTC) medications have an expectation of being safe, just because they are sold in front of the pharmacy counter rather than behind. There are potential side effects with OTC drugs, and you need to know how the OTC interacts with everything else you are taking before it can be deemed safe.

The Problem with Quack Cures

People in pain seek relief. Unfortunately, there are people who are willing and wanting to take advantage of that need. With the surge of information available on the Internet, people hawking quack cures have found it to be their playground. While there is a tremendous amount of quality health information on the Internet as well, the chore of separating good information from bad information is left to you.

Warning: Beware of Bogus Cures

You need to beware of bogus cures. However, not everyone is heeding that warning. The FDA reports that consumers respond to the pitches and spend billions of dollars a year on fraudulent health products. It's sad how sick people are preyed on for easy money, and it's even sadder that sick people are so desperate they fall for the pitch.

It's not always easy to see through quack cures, but you can develop a sixth sense about recognizing quackery. Generally speaking, quack cures sell false hope. The problem with false hope is that it distracts from real hope. Recognizing the difference will save you dollars and time otherwise wasted.

Protect yourself by remaining skeptical of treatments or purported cures which sound too good to be true. Watch out for sensational words used to promote treatment benefits such as "exclusive," "secret," "proven," "miracle," or "breakthrough." Be wary of testimonials and success stories that sound like hype and use the word *cure* or overemphasize the word *natural*. Many scams will use guarantees, whether it be guaranteed results or a money-back guarantee. They may also use claims that suggest a certain treatment is the only safe treatment or that denounce all other treatments as unsafe. Never trust treatments that are unsupported by scientific studies or claims that minimize the importance of scientific studies.

Be Logical about Quackery

Don't be led by frustration. Discuss anything you wish to add to your current treatment regimen with your doctor—your doctor must serve as your advisor. People pushing quack cures and unproven remedies can be very convincing. Beyond the possibility of wasting money and time, some of the quack treatments may be potentially harmful.

To protect yourself, make sure you consult your doctor with any information that seems questionable, do your own research by looking for more information, and be aware of the buzzwords so you're unlikely to fall victim.

Bogus or quack cures show up in likely places. Have your radar up when you are in online chat rooms, message forums, or watching infomercials. Someone wishing to tell a miraculous story can pass false hope to others. Some call those stories testimonials; others call them hogwash.

You, as a consumer, can file a complaint with the FTC at *www .ftc.gov/bcp/consumer.shtm* or with the FDA at *www.fda.gov/med watch/index.html.*

Fact

According to the Federal Trade Commission, an estimated $10 billion is spent on unproven arthritis remedies each year. One in ten people who have tried unproven arthritis remedies report harmful side effects, according to a survey by the U.S. Department of Health and Human Services. The FTC offers information on where to turn if you have questions about a product. Go to *www.ftc.gov/bcp/conline/pubs/health/whocares/arthcure.htm.*

The Benefit of Early Aggressive Treatment

Early aggressive treatment means starting stronger medications early in the course of the disease. If you have rheumatoid arthritis or one of the other types of arthritis which can cause deformity and disability, early treatment may prevent joint damage and slow disease progression. With the availability of better treatments, the prognosis is not as dismal as it was decades ago.

There are indicators that predict a more severe course of disease with rheumatoid arthritis:

- Early (i.e., younger age of) onset of severe synovitis
- Early evidence of functional limitation
- Positive test for rheumatoid factor
- Evidence of joint erosions on medical images
- Persistently elevated sedrate and CRP
- Positive test for anti-CCP
- Systemic involvement
- Family history of rheumatoid arthritis

Alert

> Joint damage in rheumatoid arthritis develops within the first two years of disease onset, possibly within the first six months in some cases. Joint damage is not always evident on x-rays early in the course of the disease; damage may have occurred before it is visible on x-rays.

Approximately 17.4 million adults in the United States with doctor-diagnosed arthritis report arthritis-attributable activity limitations, according to the Centers for Disease Control and Prevention (CDC). Of adults aged 18 to 64 with doctor-diagnosed arthritis, over 30 percent report an arthritis-attributable work limitation.

Patients with a poor prognosis can be helped by early treatment. The disease outcome in terms of severity, disability, and mortality can be impacted. Discuss your best course of treatment with your doctor. Weigh treatment benefits versus risks, and also consider potential complications of uncontrolled comorbid conditions.

Not every arthritis patient needs to be treated aggressively, and despite the recommendation for early aggressive treatment, not all patients are prescribed the more advanced medications (for example, DMARDs, biologic DMARDs) early on. Some patients may actually resist being treated with certain medications.

A study reported in the *Annals of the Rheumatic Diseases* (2006; 65:1226–1229) used a database from the Consortium of Rheumatology Researchers of North America to compare treatment plans of patients with elderly onset rheumatoid arthritis (disease onset after age sixty years) to younger-onset rheumatoid arthritis (disease onset between forty and sixty years). Study results indicated that elderly onset rheumatoid arthritis patients received combination DMARDs (disease-modifying anti-rheumatic drugs) and biologic treatments less frequently than younger-onset patients, even though both groups had identical disease duration as well as comparable disease severity and activity.

It's wise to have a conversation with your rheumatologist about your current medications and how your doctor intends to step up your treatment plan to gain better control over your symptoms. It's not uncommon for patients to feel uncertain about what's next if the medications they are on fail. If you get a sense of your doctor's thinking regarding your treatment plan, you will be able to wrap your own mind around a more aggressive treatment or using other combinations of medications.

Fact

Rheumatoid arthritis symptoms make working difficult for many people who have the disease. About 50 percent of people with rheumatoid arthritis must stop working ten to twenty years after being diagnosed. Because rheumatoid arthritis is severely disabling for many people, early aggressive treatment is your best chance for preventing disability and deformity.

Finding What Works for You

It's easy to be confused by so many treatment options. There is a lot to consider as you and your doctor try to find the right medication for you. To start, your doctor will prescribe one or more medications based on the type of arthritis you have and your level of disease activity. Beyond that, it comes down to trial and error until you establish a satisfactory response to treatment.

Arthritis is a variable disease. Patient response to arthritis treatment is also variable. When choosing a medication, any allergies you have or other medications already used to treat existing conditions should be considered. Even cost and convenience may be a factor for you.

Ask Questions about Your Medications

Asking your doctor questions about your medications will help you feel more informed about the choices being made. You should ask:

- Why your doctor chose the drug prescribed over another
- What the possible side effects are and are they common or rare side effects
- What you should do if you experience any side effects
- What tests will be routinely ordered to monitor for side effects
- When you should expect to notice some benefit from the medication

You can also discuss concerns with your pharmacist, who has vast knowledge of medications, and can also advise you on possible side effects, interactions, and other factors such as how to take your medications.

Pay Attention to Your Response

Be compliant with the dosing schedule assigned to each of your medications so that you can accurately assess their effectiveness. If you're not getting a good response, you may need to consider a medication change. Talk to your doctor.

Keep a medication diary so you can track how your medications make you feel. Always inform your doctor about any problems you are experiencing. An adjustment of dosage or a medication change may resolve the problem. Because you are the one taking the medications, you are the one who must communicate how you are responding or not responding.

By trying various drugs and making adjustments as needed, you and your doctor are trying to determine the fine line between optimal treatment and overtreatment. There are two sides to consider: Drugs have potential risks of undesirable side effects, but can also offer tremendous benefit. The possibilities become magnified when you add more medications into your treatment regimen. You must always be aware of how you react to the medications you are taking.

If you are like this, you may worry about putting chemicals into your body. The newer drugs seem to provoke more fear because they have a short track record. Doctors do their best to prescribe medications only when the benefit outweighs the potential risks. The best you can do to overcome the fear of medications is to become well informed. Ask your doctor about the drugs and do your own research. Patient education is the antidote for fearing medications.

Fact

A new report issued in September 2006 by the Institute of Medicine pointed out areas of weakness in the FDA. The main recommendations focused on improving the postapproval period (after a drug is marketed)—much more is done in the preapproval phase. The report also emphasized that approval of a drug does not mean all uncertainties about it are removed.

Fearing Addiction

Some arthritis patients who have been prescribed pain medications worry about becoming addicted. Addiction means you can't stop using the drug. According to the Mayo Clinic, people confuse addiction, tolerance, and physical dependence. If you confuse the terminology, you may fear addiction unnecessarily. Here is some clarification:

Tolerance—Occurs when your initial dose of medication is no longer achieving the same therapeutic effect it did early on. You may need your doctor to adjust your dose higher. Tolerance is considered normal and not an indication of addiction.

Physical Dependence—Your body adjusts to the drug you are taking. If you stop taking it suddenly, you may experience symptoms of withdrawal. This is physical dependence, which, once again, is not the same as addiction. With physical dependence,

L. Essential

The main categories of drugs used to treat arthritis are NSAIDs (nonsteroidal anti-inflammatory drugs), analgesics (pain medications), corticosteroids, and DMARDs (disease-modifying anti-rheumatic drugs). The newest categories of drugs are COX-2 inhibitors (a subcategory of NSAIDs) and biologic response modifiers (a subcategory of DMARDs).

Understanding Trial and Error

Before you find what works, you may have to try several medications within the same class of drugs. Though intuitively you may think all drugs in the same class are equally effective, you may experience a different response to several drugs within the same class. It may also be your experience that you have problems with one drug class but not another. It's important for you to learn about the different classes of arthritis drugs and expected response to them.

Fearing Medications

Some patients resist taking medications and prefer natural treatments. Medications are not without risk, but an overwhelming fear may interfere with the potential benefit they can provide. Without appropriate treatment, arthritis may progress with damaging consequences. A discussion with your doctor about your concerns may help allay your fears. You should be aware of the plan to monitor potential side effects and adverse reactions.

Fearing Side Effects

Some patients feel anxious, believing that medications will make them sicker than they already are. Usually, these are patients who needed no medication before.

it is possible for you to stop a drug by gradually decreasing the dose.

Addiction—You will not stop taking a drug if you are addicted, even though it has harmful effects. Addiction and physical dependence can occur simultaneously, or either one without the other.

Fear of Inadequate Regulation

The U.S. Food and Drug Administration (FDA) got a black eye a few years ago when Vioxx (an arthritis drug from the drug class known as COX-2 inhibitors) was removed from the market. Patients were left wondering what to do, and in a more general sense, what it meant about drug safety overall.

The Vioxx incident, which was the catalyst for years of legal battles still to come, left many patients distrustful of the FDA. Imagine how unsettling it is to distrust the agency responsible for the marketing of drugs which you need to improve your health.

Fear of Refractory Disease

Patients who don't show an immediate response to a new medication may start to fear they have refractory disease, meaning "hard to treat." In these cases, the patient fears the worst, loses hope, and believes they are taking the medications for no purpose since they are unable to benefit from them.

Quality of life issues counterbalance fear of medications. Consider the following:

- Do you fear becoming disabled more than you fear medications?
- Do you feel your quality of life is good and will remain good without taking medications?
- Do you fear the future and what lies ahead (e.g., losing a job, not being able to take care of yourself and your family)?
- Do you fear the future more if you are taking medications or if you are not taking medications?

Medication Side Effects Can Be Problematic

Have you ever pulled out the package insert that comes with a prescription medication? The tiny print is nearly impossible to read, yet it is packed with information about usage, contraindications (i.e., conditions which make a particular medication or treatment inadvisable), and side effects. Just because it is difficult to read does not mean you can forgo the information.

⌐ Essential

Find a resource you will use as a reference. RxList.com, The Internet Drug Index, is an example of a valuable resource with information about side effects, drug interactions, warnings, precautions, overdose information, and contraindications. Learn about each medication you take so you will be aware of any adverse events that may occur.

Side-Effect Facts

Some medication side effects are common and considered mild. Other side effects are less common and may be severe. If you're experiencing side effects, ask yourself these questions to determine severity: Are you able to continue the medication or are the side effects intolerable? Are the side effects interfering with your daily activities? Have you discussed a dosage change with your doctor? And have you tried another drug within the same class of drugs?

Remember that side effects can be temporary. Your body may respond a certain way when you first take a new drug, but may adapt later, and side effects may subside. Decide, along with your doctor, what is a reasonable amount of time to wait to see if that will happen.

Side Effects—Recognizable or Undetectable?

Side effects can be recognizable or they can be undetectable except through laboratory tests. Easily recognizable side effects include:

- Dizziness
- Drowsiness
- Upset stomach
- Diarrhea
- Constipation

- Fluid retention
- Headache
- Insomnia
- Itching
- Rash

Lab tests are used to detect some side effects, including:

- Kidney damage
- Liver damage
- Ulcers

- Anemia
- Changes in blood counts

The ability to monitor potential side effects, and the fact that changing your dosage or stopping medications can reverse some side effects, is reassuring. When deciding on a medication or whether to switch a medication, primary consideration should be given to quality of life and stabilizing disease activity.

Alert

Do not lower the dose of your medication or stop your medication without consulting your doctor. If certain drugs are stopped suddenly, there may be severe consequences. Call your doctor and find out what you should do.

The newest class of arthritis drugs, called biologic response modifiers or biologic DMARDs, is worrisome for some patients because of the possible connection to increased risk of infection and the possibility of cancer such as lymphoma. Many patients have had tremendous success with biologic DMARDs. The first of the biologics has been on the market since 1998, and was studied for several years before being marketed. Even with a favorable risk/benefit ratio, each individual patient must be vigilant about recognizing signs of adverse events and alerting their doctor.

It is important to note that any medication can cause adverse side effects at any time. It surprises many patients to learn that even if they have successfully used a medication for a period of time and responded well to it, the medication can stop working or cause undesirable side effects at any time. Any drug can become problematic at any time; monitoring drug efficacy and adverse effects is a continuous process.

When Treatments Don't Work or Stop Working

Taking medications has been compared to a roll of the dice. Not that much of a gamble really, but the point is you don't know what response you will get until you're actually using the medication.

Response to medication is individual. There are no guarantees, but just as there are side effects that may be anticipated, there are expected therapeutic responses. You must allow sufficient time to achieve the desired therapeutic effect. If you give up too soon, you may prematurely give up on a drug you shouldn't give up on. If you wait too long, you are wasting time better spent on initiating another medication or treatment.

Ⅼ Essential

Under the direction of your doctor, you should stay on a drug for a sufficient amount of time to judge its therapeutic effectiveness. When you should change depends on the drug you are taking. For example, if you do not respond to the first TNF (tumor necrosis factor) blocker after three months, switching to another will increase the chance of benefit. Even if you fail two of three TNF blockers, the third may be effective.

DMARDs (disease-modifying anti-rheumatic drugs) are slow acting and can take from one to six months to work. The biologics which includes TNF blockers may be effective in days or weeks (most often within the first month, but may take longer). Results, however, vary with the individual patient. Your individual response may be slower or faster than another patient who is receiving the same drug at the same dose.

Many patients become quite frustrated when they experience no improvement with their prescribed medication or if improvement isn't quickly apparent. It really can be a long process to find the right drug, and you may face many failed attempts before you find the right combination of drugs. Keep in mind that this is normal—most arthritis patients have failed attempts and try several drugs.

Question

What should you do after giving a medication sufficient time?
First, under the direction of your doctor, change the dose of your medication to try and elicit a better response. Second, try other drugs within the same class, if changing the dose didn't help. Third, try a drug from a different class of arthritis drugs. Finally, never give up.

Medications can be ineffective from the start or can become ineffective after being used for a period of time. Retreatment is a possibility in some situations. A study published in *Arthritis Research & Therapy* revealed that half of the study participants who used methotrexate, the most commonly prescribed DMARD for rheumatoid arthritis, found it to be ineffective at one point in the course of their treatment but benefited from the drug after being treated a second time. The finding was especially true for patients who had received a low dose during the first course of treatment with methotrexate.

However, if the biologic drug Remicade is discontinued and later restarted, there is a chance of allergic reaction. Retreatment with Remicade has caused rash, fatigue, fever, liver abnormalities, and, rarely, life-threatening allergic reactions.

Medications are just one form of arthritis treatment. Medications used in combination or medications used along with complementary treatments may elicit a better response than any single treatment used alone. If nothing seems to be working and sufficient time has been allowed, reconsider your many treatment options.

Arthritis Medications

MOST PEOPLE WITH ARTHRITIS take medications as part of their treatment regimen. Over-the-counter arthritis medications may be used or medications which must be prescribed by a doctor. The best choice of arthritis medication for an individual patient depends on the type of arthritis they have and whether their symptoms are mild, moderate, or severe. There are six major categories of drugs (also referred to as drug classes) which are used to treat the various types of arthritis.

Nonsteroidal Anti-Inflammatory Drugs (NSAIDs)

Worldwide, NSAIDs are the most commonly used class of drugs for the treatment of arthritis and have been used for more than thirty years. The two most important facts to remember about NSAIDs are that they are prescribed to treat inflammation associated with arthritis or injury to other body tissues, and as the name indicates, NSAIDs do not contain steroids.

How NSAIDs Work

NSAIDs work by inhibiting the enzyme cyclooxygenase (COX), which catalyzes arachidonic acid to prostaglandins and leukotrienes. Prostaglandins, which can be found in nearly all tissues and organs of the body, are mediators of inflammation. NSAIDs have the ability to reduce inflammation, pain, and fever.

There are two forms of cyclooxygenase, known as COX-1 and COX-2. Older, traditional NSAIDs block both COX-1 and COX-2 enzymes. A subclass of NSAIDs, called COX-2 selective inhibitors, was marketed for the treatment of arthritis in 1999. COX-2 selective inhibitors, also referred to as COX-2 inhibitors or COX-2 drugs, were developed because they were believed to have a superior gastrointestinal profile to traditional NSAIDs, which target both forms of COX. COX-1 enzyme also has a protective effect for the lining of the stomach.

Side Effects and Contraindications

There are side effects associated with NSAIDs that should not be ignored. The esophagus, small intestine, and large intestine may become irritated from NSAID use. NSAIDs can cause stomach irritation with the possibility of more serious complications including ulcers or stomach bleeding. The bleeding may occur without warning and cause death in some cases.

Pregnant women should not take NSAIDs. People who are over sixty-five years old, people who previously had a bleeding ulcer, as well as people who take blood thinners or corticosteroid medications are more at risk for developing complications.

Many doctors recommend that people who take NSAIDs also take a medication to protect the stomach. Prilosec is sold over-the-counter; your doctor can prescribe Nexium, Protonix, Prevacid, Aciphex, and Cytotec.

NSAIDs can also cause kidney problems, fluid retention, high blood pressure, heart failure, and liver problems in certain patients. Your doctor can monitor for adverse effects associated with NSAID use by performing routine blood tests. You should try to find the lowest effective dose of the NSAID you are using, as the risk of side effects will be less.

Drug Class: NSAIDs

There are some drugs that are classified as NSAIDs:

- Motrin (ibuprofen)
- Naprosyn (naproxen)
- Orudis (ketoprofen)
- Ansaid (flurbiprofen)
- Arthrotec (diclofenac sodium/misoprostal)

- Cataflam (diclofenac potassium)
- Clinoril (sulindac)
- Daypro (oxaprozin)
- Dolobid (diflunisal)
- Feldene (piroxicam)
- Indocin (indomethacin)
- Lodine (etodolac)
- Meclomen (meclofenamate sodium)
- Mobic (meloxicam)
- Nalfon (fenoprofen calcium)
- Ponstel (mefenamic acid)
- Relafen (nabumetone)
- Tolectin (tolmetin sodium)
- Voltaren (diclofenac sodium)

Salicylates are another subset of NSAIDs:

- Aspirin
- Disalcid (salsalate)
- Magnesium salsalate
- Trilisate (choline magnesium trisalicylate)

The COX-2 selective NSAIDs include:

- Celebrex
- Vioxx (no longer marketed)
- Bextra (no longer marketed)

Individual patient response to a particular NSAID can vary, making it necessary for some patients to try several different NSAIDs before determining which is most effective. NSAIDs can be taken with other arthritis medications. You can take an NSAID with a DMARD, analgesic, steroid, or biologic drug. However, you should not use two NSAIDs together.

COX-2 Inhibitors
Although COX-2 inhibitors (i.e., COX-2 selective NSAIDs) were developed for people who were at risk for developing gastrointestinal problems (including bleeding ulcers), COX-2 inhibitors didn't turn out to be more effective than traditional NSAIDs. The COX-2 drugs had the same side-effect profile as NSAIDs, as well as new side effects. With COX-2 inhibitors, especially when used at high doses, there was an

increased risk for heart attack and stroke. After further study in this area, the FDA concluded that all NSAIDs (not just the COX-2 inhibitors) could increase the risk of heart attacks or strokes. Due to the reports of heart risk associated with COX-2 inhibitors, Merck & Co. (the maker of Vioxx) voluntarily removed the drug from the market on September 30, 2004.

Bextra was the next COX-2 inhibitor to be removed from the market, on April 7, 2005. The FDA requested the removal of Bextra based on insufficient information about its cardiovascular profile. Also, there were reports of serious skin rashes associated with Bextra (perhaps Stevens-Johnson syndrome). Ultimately, in light of the risks, the FDA felt Bextra had no advantage over traditional NSAIDs in terms of pain management.

Fact

During the fifth century B.C., Hippocrates used ground willow bark to relieve arthritis aches and pains—willow bark contains salicin. By 1897, German chemist Felix Hoffman developed a treatment for his father's arthritis which became known as aspirin, the first NSAID.

The only remaining COX-2 inhibitor on the market today is Celebrex. Why did Celebrex survive but not the other COX-2 inhibitors? According to the FDA, the benefits outweighed the risks for Celebrex, so the drug was allowed to remain on the market, but it came with some requests by the FDA:

- Each Celebrex prescription was to include a patient warning regarding cardiovascular and gastrointestinal risks.
- Patients and their doctors are encouraged to discuss the risks when Celebrex is prescribed.
- Patients are advised to use the lowest effective dose of Celebrex and to use it only as long as needed.

The FDA requirements for disseminating information about risks was also added as a requirement for traditional NSAIDs, whether over-the-counter or prescribed, and changes were made to existing warning labels.

Thousands of people who took Vioxx, or who have a family member who took Vioxx, and subsequently suffered a heart attack or stroke are embroiled in a legal battle with Merck & Co. The Vioxx/Bextra debacle left arthritis patients worried and confused. Patients wondered how this could have happened. If the drugs were so unsafe, how did they ever make it to market? Most importantly, patients wondered what medications were left that were safe to take as an arthritis medication. Even though Celebrex was left on the market, patients didn't know what to trust or who to trust. Patients were encouraged, more than ever, to discuss their concerns with their doctor. Some patients stopped taking arthritis medications in search of a safer, natural treatment. Others felt comfortable sticking with Celebrex, while some patients reverted to older, traditional NSAIDs. Without question, the key is to be aware of any symptoms or side effects that seem out of the ordinary. Have routine blood tests if you take NSAIDs or COX-2 NSAIDs. Be vigilant and report anything suspicious to your doctor immediately.

Analgesics (Pain Medications)

Analgesic medications are used to treat pain, but they have no effect on inflammation or slowing disease progression. Analgesic medications work by blocking pain signals going to the brain or by interfering with the brain's interpretation of pain signals. Analgesics are divided into two categories: non-narcotics and narcotics.

Non-Narcotic Analgesics

Tylenol (acetaminophen) is the most popular and commonly used non-narcotic analgesic. Though Tylenol is considered safe and effective for mild to moderate pain, patients who use the drug on a regular basis must be mindful of the maximum allowable daily dose and recommended interval between doses. The cumulative effect of acetaminophen from the many products which contain it must also be considered by the patient. Exceeding the limits for acetaminophen can result in serious side effects, including death.

Narcotic Analgesics

Many arthritis patients use narcotic analgesics to manage severe or chronic pain associated with arthritis. While many patients find narcotic analgesics necessary for a better quality of life, others resist taking narcotic analgesics because of undesirable side effects, fear of addiction, or the stigma attached to controlled substances.

Opiates and opioids are two types of narcotic pain medications. Opioids are derivatives of opiates. Opiates are alkaloids found in opium (a liquid extract of the unripe poppy seeds). There are four classes of opioids: endogenous opioid peptides which are produced in the body (such as endorphins), opium alkaloids (such as codeine, morphine, and the baine), semisynthetic opioids (such as heroin, oxycodone, hydrocodone, dihydrocodeine, hydromorphone, oxymorphone, and nicomorphine), and fully synthetic opioids (such as Demerol, methadone, fentanyl, propoxyphene, pentazocine, buprenorphine, butorphanol, and tramadol).

There has been a push to better manage pain for patients living with chronic pain. Opioids are a common treatment for musculoskeletal pain. Poor quality of life is unacceptable for patients who could be helped by narcotic analgesics. However, you must determine for yourself how you respond to narcotic analgesics. Generally, it is now thought that people with legitimate pain don't have to fear addiction the same way a healthy person would who was abusing narcotics.

Narcotic analgesics used to treat arthritis pain include:

- Codeine (with acetaminophen, also known as Tylenol 2, 3, 4)
- Darvon (propoxyphene)
- Darvocet (propoxyphene with acetaminophen)
- MS-Contin (morphine sulfate)
- OxyContin (oxycodone)

- Percocet (oxycodone with acetaminophen)
- Percodan (oxycodone with aspirin)
- Talwin NX (pentazocine with naloxone)
- Ultram (tramadol)
- Ultracet (tramadol with acetaminophen)
- Vicodin (hydrocodone with acetaminophen)

Patients and some medical personnel sometimes refer to NSAIDs or aspirin as pain relievers, which is technically what analgesic drugs are. Though NSAIDs and aspirin do have some analgesic properties, they aren't solely analgesic drugs because they also have anti-inflammatory and antipyretic properties.

Essential

Though there are no randomized, controlled studies assessing the benefits and risks of long-term opioid use for chronic musculoskeletal conditions, there has been a shift toward accepting the use of stronger opioids to treat severe arthritis pain.

If you feel your pain is not well managed, ask your doctor about pain medications. Some patients are afraid to broach the subject with their doctor, fearing they'll be treated like a drug abuser. Discuss it! Let your doctor know how you feel about using pain medications, and at the same time, seek your doctor's opinion and advice about using pain medications.

Disease-Modifying Anti-Rheumatic Drugs (DMARDs)

Disease-modifying anti-rheumatic drugs, often referred to as DMARDs, are the second line of defense in treating rheumatoid arthritis. Years ago, DMARDs were not prescribed until it was evident that NSAIDs or a low dose of corticosteroids were not enough to slow disease progression. At that point, a DMARD was prescribed. Now, treating a rheumatoid arthritis patient aggressively in the early stages following diagnosis is thought to be important. DMARDs are now recommended early in the course of the disease in an attempt to slow disease progression.

It is possible to take more than one DMARD in certain cases, called combination therapy. Gold, penicillamine, plaquenil, sulfasalazine, and methotrexate were among the original DMARDs used to treat rheumatoid arthritis. In September 1998, another DMARD was FDA approved—Arava (leflunomide).

Gold

Gold as a treatment for arthritis was discovered by accident by a French doctor. The French doctor prescribed gold (as an injection) for a tuberculosis patient who also had arthritis. The patient received gold injections for many months as a tuberculosis treatment. The gold had an unexpected positive response for the patient's arthritis symptoms. Thereafter, gold was used to slow progression of rheumatoid arthritis. The drug could not reverse joint deformity that had already occurred though. Myochrysine (gold sodium thiomalate) and Solganol (aurothioglucose) are two forms of injectable gold salts that are available.

In 1986, gold became available in an oral formulation known as Ridaura (auranofin). About 50 percent of patients on gold had to stop using the drug due to side effects or lack of benefit. Itchy rash, mouth ulcers, and diarrhea, or loose bowels are common side effects of gold. Gold is now rarely initiated as a new therapy. At one point, gold was considered the "gold standard treatment" for moderate to severe rheumatoid arthritis; now, methotrexate is considered the gold standard treatment for rheumatoid arthritis.

Penicillamine

Penicillamine is a DMARD that became available in the 1970s. As its name suggests, the drug is somehow related to penicillin. The connection is not strong, since patients who are allergic to penicillin are still able to take penicillamine. The drug is reportedly effective in 30 percent of patients who try it.

Penicillamine is an oral drug that is initially given in low doses and built up gradually. It has similar side effects to gold, and is to be taken on an empty stomach at least one hour before meals.

Plaquenil

Originally used as a malaria treatment, plaquenil (hydroxychloroquine) is prescribed for rheumatoid arthritis patients and is also used to treat lupus. The drug is considered safe, with few side effects. An eye exam with an ophthalmologist is recommended every 6 to 12 months to check for a rare side effect which can occur with plaquenil—retinopathy. Plaquenil, which is taken orally as one or two pills a day, is effective for 30 percent of patients. It is still used by patients who for one reason or another are not candidates for some of the newer biologic DMARDs.

Sulfasalazine

Originally used to treat patients with inflammatory bowel disease, sulfasalazine has been on the market since the 1940s. Sulfasalazine (also known as azulfidine) is a combination drug of salicylate and an antibiotic. It is available as a liquid or tablet.

Sulfasalazine is used as a treatment for rheumatoid arthritis, but lost popularity because of bothersome side effects (nausea, diarrhea, vomiting, urine problems, blood diseases, and severe allergic reactions). Patients who are allergic to sulfa, aspirin, or other salicylates should not take sulfasalazine.

Methotrexate

Methotrexate was developed in the 1940s as a leukemia drug. Considered experimental in the 1970s, methotrexate was approved by the U.S. FDA to treat rheumatoid arthritis in 1988. In low doses, methotrexate is a weekly treatment for psoriatic arthritis, juvenile arthritis, vasculitis, lupus, and rheumatoid arthritis.

The usual starting dose is three to four (2.5 mg) pills a week (taken together on one day). The dose can be adjusted depending on the patient's response. Methotrexate is also available as an injectable drug, which is preferred by some patients who become nauseous or have an upset stomach after taking methotrexate tablets.

The benefit of taking methotrexate (brand names: Rheumatrex and Trexall) is usually evident in six to ten weeks for most patients. It may take twelve weeks for full benefit to be realized by some patients.

Arava

Arava is the newest of the nonbiologic DMARDs. Though Arava is thought to interfere with the formation of DNA, it's not clear how it works for rheumatoid arthritis.

Arava is usually prescribed as a 20 mg tablet to be taken once a day with food. Doctors may also prescribe a loading dose, where you initially take more of a drug for a specified period of time.

Results are slow to observe—it may take 6 to 12 weeks to notice the full benefit of using Arava. Side effects can occur: About 20 percent of patients on Arava have diarrhea. The problem can subside over time or with the help of antidiarrheal medicines. Indigestion, rash, and hair loss are also side effects of Arava, though they are less common. Abnormal liver function tests, and decreased blood cells or platelets have been observed in less than 10 percent of patients taking Arava.

Corticosteroids (Steroids)

Corticosteroids, also referred to as glucocorticoids or steroids, are drugs that are similar to cortisol, a hormone which is naturally produced in the cortex (outer layer) of the adrenal gland. These drugs are not the same as anabolic steroids that are used by some athletes to bulk up. In the 1940s, corticosteroids produced what seemed to be miraculous relief of arthritis in patients who were given daily injections. Corticosteroids were thought to be "the cure." As cortico-steroids became more widely used, it was discovered that significant side effects developed, especially at high doses or during long-term use. At low doses or for short-term use, the side effects were less severe and less evident. Currently, corticosteroids are mainly pre-scribed short-term to reduce flares of arthritis symptoms, or at a low dose that can be maintained to reduce inflammation because other medications are producing unsatisfactory results. Higher doses are used when inflammation is uncontrolled and must be quickly brought under control.

 Alert

Do not stop taking corticosteroids suddenly. The dose of corti-costeroids must be tapered gradually to allow natural cortisol production by the adrenal glands to resume. Improper steroid withdrawal can have life-threatening consequences. Talk to your doctor before you stop taking steroid medication.

How Do Corticosteroids Work?

Corticosteroids block substances or chemicals that trigger aller-gic reactions or inflammatory responses (e.g., prostaglandins). Cor-ticosteroids also interfere with the function of white blood cells that destroy foreign bodies, an important immune-system function. It is the interference with white-cell function that increases risk of infec-tion in patients taking corticosteroids.

How Are Corticosteroids Used?

Corticosteroids are used to control inflammation in types of arthritis that are characterized by joint inflammation or systemic inflammation. Among others, some of the inflammatory types of arthritis include:

- Rheumatoid arthritis
- Systemic lupus erythematosus
- Ankylosing spondylitis
- Scleroderma
- Dermatomyositis or polymyositis
- Polymyalgia rheumatica
- Vasculitis

How Are Corticosteroids Administered?

Corticosteroids used to treat arthritis can be administered four ways: Steroid pills can be taken orally; injectable forms of steroids can be given as intravenous or intramuscular injections; and topical creams or ointments which contain steroids can be applied to the skin.

Corticosteroids include:

- Deltasone (prednisone)
- Cortef (hydrocortisone)
- Cortone (cortisone)
- Medrol (methylprednisone)
- Prelone (prednisolone)
- Decadron (dexamethasone)
- Celestone (betamethasone)
- Entocort EC (budesonide)
- Kenalog (triamcinolone)

Oral prednisone is the most commonly prescribed synthetic corticosteroid to treat arthritis. Five milligrams (5 mg) of prednisone is equivalent to the body's daily production of cortisol. The other synthetic corticosteroids differ in potency and how long they stay in your system.

Biologic Response Modifiers

In 1998, the FDA approved the first of an entirely new class of drugs to treat some forms of arthritis. Referred to as biologic response modifiers, or more commonly as biologics, the drugs copy the effects of substances naturally produced by the immune system. The biologic drugs are genetically engineered, meaning human genes involved in the production of natural immune proteins in the human body are used in non-human cell cultures to produce the biologic drug.

The biologic drug can then affect certain specific immune responses, including inflammatory activity.

Current biologic drugs inhibit the actions of cytokines (proteins that serve as chemical messengers between cells). Enbrel (etanercept), Remicade (infliximab), and Humira (adalimumab) block or inhibit the action of TNF-alpha (a cytokine involved in inflammation). Kineret (anakinra) blocks interleukin-1 (IL-1), another protein that plays a role in the inflammation pathway. Orencia (abatacept) is classified as a T-cell costimulation modulator, or simply put, blocks the activation of T-cells. Rituxan (rituximab) selectively targets CD20-positive B-cells for depletion.

The language used to describe these drugs can get very technical and confusing, but the important fact to remember is that two-thirds of rheumatoid arthritis patients have a favorable response to biologics. The drugs that are believed to slow disease progression can remarkably reduce symptoms and even effect a remission in some patients.

Essential

The biologic drugs are expensive. Insurance pre-authorization is required before treatment can begin. The injectable biologic drugs are classified as specialty drugs by prescription drug plans. The biologics that are infused are considered treatments. Be sure you know your share of the cost.

How Are Biologics Different than DMARDs?

Technically speaking, the biologics are considered a subset of DMARDs in that they slow progression of the disease. Though most traditional DMARDs are taken orally, the new biologics are either injected or given intravenously. Though the biologic drugs may take weeks before any benefit is noticed by some patients, others recognize vast improvement after the first or second injection or infusion.

Enbrel—Subcutaneous (under the skin) self-injection once or twice weekly (three or four days apart).

Remicade—Intravenous (into a vein) injection over two to three hours every four to eight weeks.

Humira—Subcutaneous self-injection every other week.

Orencia—Given intravenously over thirty minutes every four weeks.

Rituxan—Intravenous infusion given twice (two weeks apart) and repeated every six to nine months. The first treatment takes six to eight hours. Subsequent treatment may be shorter or longer.

Are Biologic Drugs Suitable for Every Patient?

Biologic drugs shouldn't be used by some patients. Patients who have a previous medical history that includes recurrent infections, tuberculosis, multiple sclerosis, lymphoma, or congestive heart failure may be unsuitable candidates for the biologic drugs.

Generally, the biologic drugs are considered safe for most patients; however, a range of side effects are possible, from common side effects (injection site reactions) to more serious side effects (severe allergic reactions, increased risk of infection, increased risk of lymphoma, neurologic complications). Your doctor will consider and discuss the risk versus benefit with you.

Over-the-Counter Medications

Other than the commonly used pain-relievers aspirin and Tylenol, three of the NSAIDs are offered over-the-counter at nonprescription strength (lower strength than what is available by prescription only) for mild arthritis pain.

- Ibuprofen (brand names Advil and Motrin)
- Naproxen (brand name Aleve)
- Ketoprofen (brand names Orudis KT and Actron)

The FDA included over-the-counter, nonsteroidal anti-inflammatory medications (NSAIDs) in the revised labeling which warns of potential adverse events associated with the use of this class of drugs. It is important not to exceed the maximum allowable daily dosage and to report any gastrointestinal or cardiovascular side effects to your doctor immediately.

Other Medications

Other drugs are used to treat arthritis-related conditions. There are drugs for osteoporosis, fibromyalgia, gout, and Sjögren's syndrome, as well as medications to help with sleep problems that plague some arthritis patients.

Osteoporosis Medications

Bisphosphonates are used to treat osteoporosis (brittle bone disease). Fosamax (alendronate sodium), Actonel (risedronate sodium), and Boniva (ibandronate sodium) are the newest bisphosphonates on the market. Some are formulated to be taken weekly and some are taken once a month. Forteo (teriparatide) is given by injection. Side effects include esophagitis and the rare but potential risk of permanent damage to the jaw.

Fibromyalgia Medications

No drugs are approved specifically for fibromyalgia, but certain medications have been found to help fibromyalgia symptoms. Antidepressants such as Elavil and Endep (amitriptyline hydrochloride), Adapin and Sinequan (doxepin), or Aventyl and Pamelor (nortriptyline), and the selective serotonin reuptake inhibitors, Prozac (fluoxetine), Paxil (paroxetine), and Zoloft (sertraline) may help fibromyalgia patients relax and get deep, restful sleep.

Muscle relaxers, such as Flexeril, Soma, Robaxin, or Skelaxin, are often prescribed to ease muscular aches and pains associated with fibromyalgia and all types of arthritis. Neurontin (gabapentin) or Lyrica (pregabalin), classified as anti-seizure medications, can also help with pain, sleep problems, and the restless leg syndrome affecting some fibromyalgia patients.

Pain associated with arthritis can be exacerbated by lack of sleep. If you have difficulty falling asleep, ask your doctor about sleep medications. There are several to choose from—Ambien, Restoril, Rozerem, Sonata, and Lunesta—which will promote restful sleep.

 Alert

> Only take sleep medications as directed. You may have a particularly bad night trying to get to sleep, but if you have taken your Ambien (or other sleep medication), that's all you're allowed for twenty-four hours. If you still can't sleep after taking medication, get out of bed, do something relaxing, and then try going back to bed.

Gout Medications

Several medications help gout patients control uric-acid levels. Allopurinol and probenecid are prescribed for patients who produce too much uric acid. Another drug, colchicine, is prescribed to prevent or ease gout attacks.

Sjögren's Syndrome Medications

Sjögren's Syndrome is an arthritis-related condition characterized by dry eyes and dry mouth. Evoxac (cevimeline) is a drug prescribed to help with dry mouth. Salagen (pilocarpine) tablets are also used to treat dry mouth associated with Sjögren's syndrome. Restasis (cyclosporine) is a drug used to treat chronic dry eye conditions.

CHAPTER 8

Other Treatment Options

THOUGH MEDICATIONS ARE THE MOST COMMONLY USED and often the first-tried treatments for arthritis, there are other options. Whether other treatments are used because medications produce an unsatisfactory response, or as an adjunct therapy, it's important to know all of your options. Arthritis is a chronic, progressive disease. As your condition progresses, your treatment plan may be altered to control new symptoms. Treatments may be considered to prevent further damage caused by arthritis or to repair damage already done.

Viscosupplementation

Viscosupplementation is a procedure that involves injecting a thick, gel-like substance (hyaluronate) into the joint. The procedure is approved for the treatment of osteoarthritis of the knee. It's also being studied as a treatment for the hip, shoulder, and ankle. Hyaluronate injections are considered treatments, not drugs. With osteoarthritis, the cartilage of a joint breaks down or wears away. There is also loss of joint lubrication, which normally makes a joint glide with ease, as synovial fluid loses its viscosity (i.e., thickness, stickiness, consistency). The loss of lubrication contributes to joint pain, stiffness, and limited mobility. Normal synovial fluid contains hyaluronic acid. Viscosupplementation was developed as a way to improve the lubrication of synovial fluid, reduce pain associated with osteoarthritis, and improve a patient's level of activity and function.

Availability of Viscosupplementation Products

In the United States, the FDA approved viscosupplementation in 1997 for osteoarthritis of the knee. The procedure had already been used in Asia and Europe for several years. Currently, there are five hyaluronic-acid based products (hyaluronates) used for viscosupplementation, which are listed below in the order the FDA approved them:

- Hyalgan (5/28/1997)
- Synvisc (8/8/1997)
- Supartz (1/24/2001)
- Orthovisc (2/5/2004)
- Euflexxa (12/3/2004)

When Is Viscosupplementation an Appropriate Treatment?

Generally speaking, as with any treatment, the result of viscosupplementation is likely better before severe damage has been done. The procedure is usually used after patients have tried and failed other treatment options.

The injections, which go directly into your knee joint, can be given in one or both knees at the same time. If there is fluid around your knee joint, your doctor can remove it at the same time as the injection using the same needle stick. Synvisc, Orthovisc, and Euflexxa are injected weekly for three weeks. Hyalgan and Supartz are injected weekly for five weeks.

Alert

The FDA has classified viscosupplements as devices, not as drugs. Various medical insurance plans differ in how they cover viscosupplantation. Be sure to check and see if it's covered by your plan, and if so, how many treatments will be covered.

Has Viscosupplementation Been Proven Effective?

Studies have tried to ascertain the effectiveness of viscosupplementation for mild or moderate osteoarthritis, compared to corticosteroid injection or NSAIDs. The results are inconclusive. At best, it was concluded that of the patients who did obtain pain relief from the procedure, most found the relief to occur eight to twelve weeks after initial treatment. Some resources pitched viscosupplementation as a way to delay joint replacement surgery. However, there has been no conclusive evidence that viscosupplementation delays or halts the disease course of osteoarthritis. The procedure is not a cure for osteoarthritis and is not approved for rheumatoid arthritis.

Important Things to Know about Viscosupplementation

There are important facts you should know about viscosupplementation. The benefit of viscosupplementation is a long-term effect—it starts weeks or months after injection and lasts for several months—so don't expect to notice immediate pain relief following treatment. You may have a local reaction at the injection site; applying ice should help with any minor pain or swelling.

It is recommended that you not engage in strenuous activity or unnecessary or excessive weight bearing on the leg for forty-eight hours after the injection. If you have an allergy to eggs or poultry, be sure to tell your doctor. Some, but not all, of the products used for viscosupplementation are made from rooster combs.

Prosorba Column

The Prosorba Column, also known as Protein-A Immunoadsorption Therapy, is a plastic cylinder containing a sand-like substance coated with a special material called protein A. It was FDA approved in March of 1999 for the treatment of rheumatoid arthritis. The Prosorba Column had been approved in 1987 to treat idiopathic thrombocytopenic purpura.

The cylinder is used with a procedure known as apheresis. Blood is drawn from your arm and passes through a machine that separates plasma from blood cells. The plasma passes through the Prosorba Column, where antibodies (which play a role in rheumatoid arthritis) are removed. The plasma which has the antibodies removed and the blood cells are mixed back together and returned to the patient through a vein in the opposite arm.

Usual Course of Prosorba

Prosorba treatment is rarely used, but when it is, the usual course of treatment involves twelve weekly outpatient sessions that take approximately two hours. It is only considered for patients with moderate to severe rheumatoid arthritis who have failed DMARDs or biologics.

In clinical trials, 30 percent to 40 percent of patients benefited from the Prosorba Column and some achieved remission that lasted for a year or longer.

 Alert

The Prosorba Column procedure is contraindicated in patients taking ACE inhibitors for blood pressure or heart disease unless the patient undergoes a seventy-two-hour withdrawal period for the ACE inhibitor. Discuss it with your doctor if you take an ACE inhibitor.

Cost and Insurance Coverage

The procedure is classified as a medical device, not a drug. Medicare covers the procedure for severe rheumatoid arthritis patients with active disease, which is defined as having: more than five swollen joints, more than twenty tender joints, and morning stiffness lasting more than one hour. In order to be covered by Medicare, patients also must have failed three or more DMARDs. Failure is specified as an insufficient response, not as intolerance. Medicaid and most private insurance companies cover the procedure, but may have some restrictions. As always, you should check with your own insurance to be certain. The twelve-week course of Prosorba carries a hefty price tag of $18,000 or more.

What Else Should You Know about Prosorba?

Prosorba is not as well-known as other rheumatoid arthritis treatments. Here are some other important facts you should know before being treated with Prosorba:

- Some patients who responded to the Prosorba Column noticed results after six weeks, while others took more than twenty weeks.
- Twenty minutes prior to Prosorba treatment, you should do arm bends using one pound hand weights, use a rubber ball to perform hand squeezes, or apply heat to promote circulation.
- Drink plenty of fluids (caffeine free) the day before and day of treatment with Prosorba.
- The veins used for the Prosorba treatment should not be used for blood drawing during the course of the twelve-week treatment.

It is not unusual for you to feel flu-like symptoms after treatment, but usually the symptoms are mild and temporary. Patients also report having symptoms like an arthritis flare after treatment (such as fatigue, joint pain, and swelling). Patients with a past history of infection or blood clotting problems need to mention that to their doctor. Patients with severe heart or lung disease or who have had recent surgery may not be candidates for Prosorba.

Topical Medications

Not every treatment for arthritis is a pill or an injection. There are creams, gels, ointments, balms, and lotions that can be rubbed into the skin over the affected joint. Some help to relieve pain, while others work on inflammation.

Fact

The American College of Rheumatology acknowledges the role of topical agents in the treatment guidelines for osteoarthritis. Patients who have mild pain, but do not get enough help from Tylenol alone, may be candidates for topical medications.

The topical products are available over-the-counter and have one or more active ingredients. By rubbing into the joint locally, topical products have less risk for systemic side effects.

Topical Counterirritants

Counterirritants stimulate or irritate the nerve endings to distract the brain and take attention off of musculoskeletal pain. Menthol, oil of wintergreen, camphor, eucalyptus oil, turpentine oil, dihydrochloride, and methyl nicotinate are ingredients found in the brand-name products ArthriCare, Eucalyptamint, Icy Hot, and Therapeutic Mineral Ice.

Topical Capsaicin

Capsaicin works by depleting the amount of a neurotransmitter called substance P that sends pain messages to the brain. Capsaicin is a highly purified product derived from cayenne peppers. Burning or stinging may be noticed with initial use. Topical products that contain capsaicin are sold as Zostrix or Zostrix HP and Capzasin-P, among others. It is very important to avoid the eyes because topical capsaicin can cause burning.

Topical Salicylates

Salicylate topical products work as oral salicylates do—by inhibiting prostaglandins. They also work as counterirritants. Topical salicylates are sold under the names Aspercreme, BENGAY, Flexall, Mobisyl, and Sportscreme.

Topical NSAIDs

Topical NSAIDs contain diclofenac and are sold in some countries as Pennsaid lotion. Research has shown the benefit of topical NSAIDs to be short-lived. In one study, topical NSAIDS offered better pain relief than the dummy treatment for the first two weeks, after which it was no more effective than the dummy treatment. Topical NSAIDS were less effective than comparable oral NSAIDS, even in the first two weeks. Local compounding of the agent at a higher dose may increase efficacy.

Topical Agents with MSM or Glucosamine

MSM and glucosamine, besides being dietary supplements, are found in topical creams and gels. There have yet to be studies that prove their effectiveness when compared to oral MSM and oral glucosamine.

Before trying topical agents, talk to your doctor. Discuss whether they are safe for you to use. Also inquire whether you should continue using them past a certain point if benefit is not noticeable. Ask which topical agent your doctor would recommend, as well as questions about how and when to apply the topical preparation. It's your decision and your money, but a well-informed decision is best.

Clearly, the best candidates for topical medications are those patients who are unable to take oral medications for one reason or another; it may be worth a trial in such cases. There is no cure for arthritis in a tube of cream. You are aiming for mild pain relief at best. Don't write it off as nothing until you try the products, but at the same time don't hope for too much.

Surgical Options

Patients who have severe joint damage that is painful and interferes with daily activities may be candidates for surgery. The goal of surgery is to repair the damage, reduce pain, and restore function. Joint surgery should not be performed for cosmetic purposes alone.

Depending on the joint involved and the soft-tissue impact, there are several orthopedic surgery options to repair joint damage, including total joint replacement, arthrodesis (fusion), synovectomy, arthroscopy, osteotomy, and resection.

Joint Replacement

Total joint replacement surgery is commonly performed on the hips (THR) and knees (TKR). Other joints, including the shoulders, elbows, ankles, and knuckles may also be replaced. With a total joint replacement (also referred to as arthroplasty), the damaged joint is removed and replaced with a prosthesis made of metal, ceramic, or plastic. Some prostheses are cemented and others are uncemented. The uncemented type of prosthesis is designed to allow bone to grow into the porous coating on the prosthesis and stabilize the joint.

L. Essential

Some patients are told by their doctors that they are too young for joint replacement surgery. Future revisions, which become increasingly more difficult and complicated, are the reason for the age issue. However, it's also a quality of life issue. Be open with your doctor and offer your opinions about joint surgery.

Over the years, there have been advancements in the field of reconstructive joint surgery. Advancements, such as minimally invasive surgery, have made joint replacement recovery easier for patients. The minimally invasive procedure requires less dissection and smaller incisions for patients who qualify for the procedure. Another significant advancement has been the development of the unicondylar knee replacement or partial knee replacement. The knee joint is comprised of the medial, lateral, and kneecap compartment. When only the medial or lateral component is severely affected by arthritis, there are distinct advantages to the unicondylar knee replacement over a total knee replacement. Because the surgeon is dealing with only one component, there is less bone loss. If the need for revision arises, the procedure is easier for the surgeon to perform and recovery is shorter for the patient.

Joint replacements can last decades in some patients. At some point, the prosthesis can wear out and revision surgery is required for that joint. Loosening is a common problem with hip replacements. Some designs that have a plastic liner in the acetabular component shed microscopic fragments due to the friction caused by walking and everyday use of the joint. The fragments can cause an inflammatory process and the end result is a loose hip replacement. Loose hip prostheses are very painful and range of motion can be severely impacted.

A revision is a repeat total joint replacement, but first the old prosthesis has to come out. The revision is considered more difficult than a virgin (first-time) hip replacement, and takes longer. If you need a revision, it is very important to have a surgeon who is experienced with revision joint surgery.

Gender-specific knee replacements have been another interesting development in joint surgery. More than 400,000 knee replacements are performed in the United States every year. Two-thirds of the knee replacement patients are women. Though traditional knee replacement prostheses come in various sizes, a new prosthesis developed by Zimmer is gender-specific, designed just for women. The reason for the gender-specific knee is that women's knees are shaped differently than men's knees. The expectation is that the gender-specific knee will perform better—time will tell.

Hip Resurfacing

As an alternative to total joint replacement, another procedure known as resurfacing may be an option for some patients. The Birmingham Hip Resurfacing System is the only FDA-approved hip resurfacing system available in the United States. The system was first introduced in the United Kingdom in 1997 and has been used in other countries.

The Birmingham hip is a two component, metal-on-metal prosthesis. A metal cup fits into the acetabulum after it's resurfaced, and another metal cup fits over the femoral ball after it's resurfaced. The benefit of the Birmingham hip, which has been implanted in more than 60,000 patients, is that it conserves more bone than a traditional hip replacement, and it preserves future surgical options, especially for younger patients who may face more revisions.

Arthrodesis

Arthrodesis is the technical name for joint fusion. Arthrodesis is performed for one purpose—to relieve pain. The procedure can be performed on ankles, wrists, fingers, and thumbs. With arthrodesis, the two bones that form a joint are joined or fused together. Mobility and flexibility is lost following a fusion, but the joint is more stable and stronger and pain relief can be as much as 100 percent. After the procedure, if performed on your ankle, you will likely be non-weight-bearing for several weeks or months until x-rays reveal the bones are fusing. Other joints that are being fused (such as wrist, fingers, thumbs) may be splinted or casted to keep a patient from moving or using the joint until it shows x-ray evidence of fusion.

Arthroscopy

Arthroscopy is both a diagnostic procedure and a surgical procedure. An arthroscope (thin tube with a light at the end) is inserted directly into a joint through a small incision. The arthroscope is hooked up to a closed-circuit television and the surgeon can view the joint damage and decide what repairs can be performed arthroscopically to relieve pain. Arthroscopic surgery is most commonly performed on knees and shoulders.

Synovectomy, Osteotomy, and Resection

Synovectomy can be performed by surgically opening the knee or as an arthroscopic procedure. During a synovectomy, the synovium or lining of the joints is removed. A synovectomy can reduce joint pain and swelling associated with rheumatoid arthritis and is thought to slow joint destruction. It's not a one-time fix, however; the synovium often grows back.

An osteotomy involves the cutting and repositioning of bone. The procedure is primarily used for patients with mild osteoarthritis who have misalignment of a joint. Osteotomy is used to shorten, lengthen, or correct misalignment of bone.

A surgical resection involves removing part or all of a bone. Most commonly, resection is performed on the feet (metatarsal resection, bunion removal) because pain is so severe it interferes with walking. The recovery period can take time, but the goal is to regain a certain level of comfort.

Physical Therapy and Occupational Therapy

You likely keep an eye out for the mention of a new medication, dietary supplement, or treatment that may relieve arthritis symptoms more effectively than whatever you're currently taking. Don't overlook other ways you can help manage the disease. Physical therapy and occupational therapy are two avenues that can also help control pain and maintain joint function.

If your doctor has not recommended physical therapy or occupational therapy to you, bring up the possibility and see if your doctor feels you could benefit from one or more sessions. In some states, a patient can self-refer to a physical therapist, while in other states a doctor's referral is required. As with any treatment, be sure you are familiar with how your insurance covers physical therapy evaluations and sessions.

Physical Therapy as Part of Arthritis Management

Generally, physical therapy focuses on an individual patient's physical and functional status. Mobility, posture, and body mechanics are carefully assessed by a physical therapist before recommendations are made. Therapeutic exercises are prescribed, which are chosen to improve strength and stamina.

It is important for you to be evaluated by a physical therapist before starting an exercise program. A therapist can assess your needs and modify exercises to suit you specifically. If you are exercising improperly, you can do more damage than if you were not exercising at all. The advice of a professional is valuable. The therapist may also recommend heat, cold, hydrotherapy, or electrical stimulation to be used before, during, or after exercise.

By assessing your physical limitations and increasing your activity level to what is tolerable for you, preserving your independence becomes another goal of physical therapy. Besides exercise to improve or preserve the range of motion of your joints, physical therapists can recommend mobility aids or adaptive equipment or recommend a consultation with an occupational therapist who works extensively with adaptive equipment.

Occupational Therapy as Part of Arthritis Management

An occupational therapist focuses on everyday tasks of daily living. Occupational therapy emphasizes joint protection techniques and proper body mechanics in terms of daily activities. Any movement should be done in ways that are optimal for minimizing stress on your joints. This includes getting in and out of a chair or bed, getting in and out of a car, getting on and off of the toilet, and lifting, bending, reaching, and gripping.

Occupational therapists focus on improving your ability to perform daily activities, and also help you adapt when functional ability is impaired. An occupational therapist will assess your home and work environment to be sure they are helping you maintain your ability to function in those settings.

Occupational therapists, as well as physical therapists, are licensed professionals who are an integral part of a patient's health-care team. They are trained to assess and evaluate a patient's individual abilities through interview, observation, and formal assessment for the purpose of setting goals and tracking progress.

Question

If your doctor hasn't recommended physical therapy or occupational therapy, should you assume it's unimportant?
Not necessarily. When you see your doctor, time is limited. Your doctor bases decisions and recommendations on his findings as well as what you disclose. If arthritis is affecting your daily activities, tell your doctor.

Orthotics

Orthotics (splints, braces, and insoles) can decrease pain in the foot, knee, hip, ankle, and lower back. Orthotics support muscles, tendons, ligaments, and bone to add stability. There are rigid, soft, or semirigid orthotic devices. Rigid orthotics are made of plastic or another hard material to prevent movement in a joint that is functioning abnormally. Soft orthotics are primarily used to take pressure off of sore spots or absorb shock. Semirigid orthotics are used to position a joint and improve balance.

To evaluate the success of using an orthosis, the Cochrane Group analyzed four studies involving 440 people with osteoarthritis of the knee.

One of the studies compared patients who wore a valgus knee brace to correct outward turning of the knee to those who wore a neoprene sleeve, versus no support, for a period of six months. People who wore the brace improved the most with regard to pain, stiffness, and physical function.

A second study concluded that wearing wedged insoles, whether neutrally or laterally, decreased pain and stiffness after six months.

The third study compared a strapped insole to a laterally wedged insole. A laterally wedged insole is thinner at the instep and thicker at the outside of the foot. The strapped insole decreased pain, while the laterally wedged sole did not decrease pain. Both the strapped insole and laterally wedged sole improved function, however.

Fact

A rigid orthosis is often tried before ankle arthrodesis or fusion is performed. The orthosis can promote natural fusion in some cases, but also gives a patient a good idea of what the joint will feel like after surgical fusion.

The fourth study showed that a strapped insole decreased pain, but a sock-type insole did not decrease pain in the osteoarthritis patients.

There are many designs of orthotics, and custom-designed orthotics may be appropriate for some patients. It may take a trial of different types of orthotics and the advice of an orthotics specialist to determine what is best for you if an orthotic is indicated.

CHAPTER 9
Alternative or Complementary Treatments

ALTERNATIVE OR COMPLEMENTARY TREATMENTS have become increasingly popular among arthritis patients. Some patients seek out alternative treatments because conventional treatment is not producing satisfactory results. Other reasons include a fear of side effects from prescription medications, a belief that natural treatments are safer, and a desire to find more effective ways to cope with chronic pain. Patients are not advised to forgo conventional treatment in favor of alternative treatment. New terminology has cropped up to represent the use of both conventional and alternative treatments—alternative medicine, complementary medicine, or integrative medicine.

Massage Therapy

Massage is an increasingly popular way to relieve arthritis pain, but it's not a new concept. Hippocrates wrote over 2,000 years ago that doctors should be adept at "rubbing that can bind a joint that is loose and loosen a joint that is too hard."

Massage therapy can improve joint mobility, relieve muscle tension, and stimulate blood flow to the tissues. Beyond that, anyone who has had a massage will tell you that the greatest benefit is the relaxation it brings. A therapeutic massage performed by a trained massage therapist involves hands-on manipulation of soft tissues by rubbing, stroking in specific motions, and applying pressure. There are many types of massage, including:

Swedish massage—Stroking and kneading on top of muscles and gently moving joints throughout the whole body.

Deep-tissue massage—Slow strokes and intense pressure on the deep layers of muscle. This can cause soreness and may not be appropriate for every arthritis patient.

Myofascial release—Long strokes to relieve tension in the connective tissue around muscles.

Trigger-point therapy—Finger pressure to points of the body that are knotted or tense, or at specific points that can trigger pain in the body.

Acupressure (an Asian technique)—Finger pressure at the specific points used for acupuncture. Acupressure unblocks the flow of life energy called qi.

The best way to learn and experience massage is to find a therapist who is nationally certified in therapeutic massage and bodywork and a graduate of a training program accredited by the Commission on Massage Therapy Accreditation.

Essential

Having the right massage therapist can make the difference between a good and bad experience. To find a qualified therapist in your local area, go to, ✑www.amtamassage.org or call, 888-843-2682.

It is your responsibility to interview your massage therapist, just as the therapist will be interviewing you. Ask if the therapist has experience working with people who have arthritis. Ask how your therapist expects that you will benefit from massage, and also ask about her approach.

Massage therapy sessions usually last an hour to an hour and a half, but the session can be modified for you if needed. Four to six weekly sessions are needed before you will notice improvement. The cost for a massage therapy appointment has a wide range, from $30 to over $100 per hour. Check with your insurance; it may be covered if your doctor prescribes massage for you.

Acupuncture

Started 2,000 years ago in China, and practiced throughout Asia and Europe, acupuncture is gaining popularity in the United States. If you learn about the background or history of acupuncture, you will find that traditional Chinese medicine is based on an essential life force (called qi) which flows through the body along meridians (like channels). The meridians serve to irrigate the body and provide nourishment to tissues.

If there is an obstruction to the meridian, qi is blocked and pain and disease are the result.

Fact

With acupuncture, very thin needles are inserted into specific points along the meridian in an effort to unblock the energy channel. There are about 2,000 points on the body that can be used for acupuncture.

Along with the needles, some practitioners use heat, friction, or electrical impulses. Electroacupuncture is a form of acupuncture whereby the needles are attached to a device that generates an electric pulse and creates a small current between pairs of needles.

Where Are the Meridians?

Western researchers have not confirmed that the meridians exist. The meridians are said to not correspond with circulatory or nerve pathways of the body. Just because western researchers have not found the meridians, does not mean that the benefits patients have experienced from acupuncture are not real. Several studies were run, some too small, others poorly designed, but still the NIH concluded that acupuncture may be useful for osteoarthritis.

Acupuncture Sessions—What to Expect

Expect to stay for one and one-half hours for your initial acupuncture session. Subsequent sessions are usually shorter, taking thirty to sixty minutes. Usually to start, three to fifteen needles are placed and left for several minutes. The number of sessions will depend on the severity of your arthritis. The cost for an acupuncture session ranges from $30 to more than $100. Your insurance may cover acupuncture for arthritis. For referrals to qualified physicians trained in acupuncture, go to *www.medicalacupuncture.org*. If you intend to use an acupuncturist who is not a doctor, choose one who is certified or licensed.

Biofeedback

Biofeedback is a technique that promotes relaxation and imagery to control body functions such as breathing, heart rate, blood pressure, skin temperature, muscle tension, and pain. The setup for biofeedback has you connected to electrodes to measure body functions that are displayed on a monitor you can watch. Three common types of biofeedback include electromyography, to measure muscle tension; thermal biofeedback, to measure skin temperature; and electroencephalography, to measure brain activity.

Essential

Each biofeedback session lasts less than one hour. The number of sessions depends on the condition being treated. Most patients notice benefit after eight to ten sessions. It's not a quick fix, and it takes a commitment on the part of the patient.

Your biofeedback practitioner will evoke stress in you and then guide you to relax—all while you're observing the monitor and recognizing how stress versus relaxation changes the parameters on the monitor. From the biofeedback experience, you're taught to control your own body functions.

Goals of Biofeedback

The goal of biofeedback is that you learn to control body functions when not attached to the monitor as well as when you are attached to the monitor. The benefit of biofeedback is being able to use the principles in the practical world. Research has shown that biofeedback is especially helpful for neck and shoulder pain and Raynaud's disease. Biofeedback hasn't been found to help lower-back pain as much.

Licensed Practitioner

Most states don't restrict who can offer biofeedback services. The Association for Applied Psychophysiology and Biofeedback (AAPB) emphasizes at *www.aapb.org* that anyone providing biofeedback services should be certified by the Biofeedback Certification Institute of America. Be cautious about biofeedback practitioners who are not certified, especially in a clinical setting.

Success of Biofeedback

According to AAPB, several studies (some small controlled studies and small clinical studies) indicated that study participants had decreases in pain and physical markers of arthritis following temperature and muscle tension biofeedback. The therapy was rated 3 for efficacy on a scale of 1 to 5.

Essentially, as described by the Mayo Clinic, biofeedback uses your mind to control your body. It's a high-tech way of using your mind to improve your health, which in the case of arthritis patients means using your mind to control pain, muscle tension, and fatigue. Because practitioners aren't sure exactly how biofeedback works other than theoretically, you are not advised to stop conventional treatments when participating in biofeedback.

Music Therapy

Music therapy is the clinical use of music to achieve individualized goals such as healing, pain relief, and relaxation under the guidance of a certified, professional music therapist. Trained to assess the emotional and physical health of the individual patient through response to music, a music therapist designs music sessions which include music improvisation, music listening, song writing, lyric discussions, music and imagery, and music performance.

Music therapy, which sounds very new age, is anything but a new therapeutic concept. According to the American Music Therapy Association, the notion that music could affect healing has been around since the writings of Aristotle and Plato. In more modern times, amateur and professional musicians used to entertain patients in the Veterans Administration hospitals following both World War I and World War II. The response of patients, both physically and emotionally, led to the hiring of musicians by hospitals. In 1944, born of the need for music therapists, the first college curriculum for a music degree was started at Michigan State University. Music therapists must complete the college curriculum, intern, and pass the national examination from the Certification Board for Music Therapists.

Music Therapy Misconceptions

There are several misconceptions about music therapy. Contrary to what some people think, patients do not have to have musical ability to benefit from music therapy; any style of music, not just soft music (for example, dentist-office music, elevator music), can be used for music therapy, and not only people with health problems benefit from music therapy. Healthy individuals use it to relieve stress and exercise.

Is Music Therapy Covered by Insurance?

According to the American Music Therapy Association, Medicare will cover music therapy if a doctor prescribes the therapy for a patient, if it is considered necessary for the treatment plan, is based on a documented treatment plan, and providing the patient shows some level of improvement.

Medicaid coverage varies by state. The only way to know for sure is to check with your state's Medicaid office. Similarly, if you have private insurance, you must check with your specific insurer. Some insurers cover music therapy on a case-by-case basis, after assessing the medical necessity. It has been estimated that approximately 20 percent of music therapists receive third-party reimbursement.

Fact

The American Music Therapy Association was founded in 1998 and represents over 5,000 music therapists. The association was preceded by the National Association for Music Therapy in 1950 and the American Association for Music Therapy in 1971. Their goal is to develop the therapeutic use of music.

Does Music Therapy Work?

Results from a small study involving sixty patients who had continuous pain from osteoarthritis, rheumatoid arthritis, or disc problems showed that music therapy eased the perception of chronic pain. Researchers from the Cleveland Clinic divided study participants into two groups: One group listened to music for one hour a day (half chose their own music while the other half chose from five selections) and the second group did not listen to music. There was a significant reduction in pain and in depression associated with pain for the group who listened to music, whether it was their selection or selected from the limited list.

Meditation/Relaxation

Research has shown that meditation helps relieve symptoms associated with arthritis including pain, stress, anxiety, and fatigue. Some studies suggest the meditation may work toward balancing the immune system and promoting healing.

Meditation techniques are geared toward quieting the mind as well as relaxing the whole body. There are many meditation techniques or types of meditation. Some, but not all, are associated with religion and spirituality.

Mindfulness meditation (also referred to as Vipassana meditation) focuses completely on your breathing. It may be helpful to take deep breaths when practicing mindfulness meditation, but not necessarily. It is important to breathe in slowly, hold, and breathe out slowly. You may find it's not quite as easy as it sounds because your mind will start to wander. When that happens, refocus on your breathing; the goal of mindfulness meditation is to remain in the moment and be aware of what you are doing at any particular moment.

Transcendental meditation is another well-known meditation technique. With transcendental meditation, a mantra or holy phrase is repeated over and over to allow thoughts and feelings that develop to pass by and not be distracting.

Researching Meditation and Health Benefits

Major universities have studied the stress management and health benefits associated with meditation. Though there have been hundreds of studies, not many focused on the effect of meditation on arthritis symptoms. Several studies did specifically show that meditation was effective for fibromyalgia patients by affecting pain, fatigue, and sleep disturbance.

Stress has been associated with the flaring of arthritis symptoms. Meditation alone or in combination with other relaxation techniques (yoga, Tai Chi, etc.) helps to manage stress. Meditation has also been shown to affect other physical parameters, including heart rate, blood pressure, cortisol level, brain activity on MRI, and possibly immune function. More research is needed to find answers to still-puzzling questions: Why doesn't every patient benefit from meditation? Does meditation only help highly motivated patients?

It's definitely worth a trial, but patients are advised not to give up their conventional treatment when they begin meditation, or even after experiencing some improvement in symptoms.

Alert

Don't give up because you lose concentration. Results will not be immediate; mindfulness meditation takes practice. *The Arthritis Helpbook* by Kate Lorig, R.N., Ph.D. and James F. Fries, M.D. suggests practicing mindfulness meditation for fifteen to thirty minutes a day, four or five times a week.

Chiropractic

Chiropractic treatment uses hands-on manipulation and adjustment to relieve pressure on nerves caused by misalignment of the body structures. Chiropractic is based on the theory that the nervous system controls all body functions and that abnormal nerve function results in disease. Manipulation and adjustment is performed to correct alignment abnormalities that cause impaired nerve function.

Doctors of Chiropractic

Not all Doctors of Chiropractic (DC) have the same education or practice the same way. The minimum education required to become a Doctor of Chiropractic is two years of college, followed by four years in a school of chiropractic medicine. Passing a national-board examination and becoming state-licensed is required to practice.

Some chiropractors only practice spinal manipulation, while others practice spinal manipulation and recommend other treatments too, which may include physical therapy, counseling, and nutritional advice. The former are affiliated with the International Chiropractors Association (*www.chiropractic.org*), while the latter are affiliated with the American Chiropractic Association (*www.amerchiro.org*).

There are over 60,000 Doctors of Chiropractic in the United States with active licenses to practice.

Spinal manipulation is not recommended for patients with rheumatoid arthritis of the neck. Even for others, a cervical x-ray should precede spinal manipulation.

Question

Is spinal manipulation a modern treatment or healing practice?
Spinal manipulation is considered one of the oldest healing practices: It was described by Hippocrates in ancient Greece. The modern profession of chiropractic was founded in 1895 by Daniel David Palmer. Since then, different approaches to chiropractic have developed.

Popular Alternative

According to the American Chiropractic Association, approximately 7.4 percent of the population used chiropractic care in 2002 (the last available statistics). The percentage was higher than yoga, massage, acupuncture, or diet-based treatment. National surveys have revealed that patients prefer chiropractic treatment to medical care for back and neck pain, but that includes all causes of back and neck pain.

For arthritis, studies are often small. One study, several years old, is still frequently referred to if you search for information about chiropractic treatment for arthritis. The study found that of more than 200 patients who responded to a survey, 63 percent who visited a rheumatologist for osteoarthritis, rheumatoid arthritis, or fibromyalgia also tried some type of alternative or complementary treatment. Chiropractic was the most used alternative treatment, with 31 percent of respondents having tried it at least once. Among forms of alternative treatment that were regularly used, chiropractic placed second behind herbal remedies, and was followed by copper bracelets and magnets, electric stimulators, and dietary supplements. Of the patients who tried chiropractic treatment, 73 percent said it was helpful. Only

45 percent had told their doctors about using an alternative treatment, but 71 percent of the rheumatologists approved of it.

Reasons given for using chiropractic care or other alternative treatments were what you might expect: to control pain, heard it would help, it's considered safe, a family member or friend was helped by it, and prescription medications are not working.

However, since this popular study was reported, many new arthritis drugs have been approved and marketed, including the biologics. It is possible that the percentages have shifted and that patient satisfaction with prescription medications and conventional treatments has improved. If you aren't satisfied with your conventional treatment, discuss chiropractic care with your rheumatologist.

Copper Bracelets

You will see copper bracelets sold on the Internet by myriad online stores, but you will come up short on evidence that they work to relieve arthritis symptoms; you will only find personal testimonials.

Alert

Copper bracelets definitely fall under the category of unproven remedy. Don't be lured into spending a lot of money and putting faith in a treatment which has no basis; approach the myth of copper bracelets with a skeptical eye.

The practice of wearing copper bracelets began about a century ago when people who wore copper bracelets claimed their arthritis symptoms were relieved. There was no scientific evidence to support that the improvement was anything but normal fluctuation of arthritis symptoms. The placebo effect is also a possible explanation, as it is with all unproven treatments.

There are many theories about how copper bracelets may work. The most common theory suggests that copper salts have antioxidant properties that may prevent free radicals from damaging your joints. Theoretically, copper salts are absorbed through the skin from the copper bracelet or other copper jewelry. However, skin is unable to absorb the amount of copper salts from a copper bracelet that would be needed to prevent damage caused by free radicals. Beyond that, many copper bracelets have a lacquer applied to prevent tarnish. The lacquer would interfere with copper absorption as well.

Magnet Therapy

Magnets produce a type of energy known as a magnetic field. There are two types of magnets: static and electromagnetic. Static magnets, which are the most commonly marketed magnets touted to have health benefits, produce an unchanging magnetic field. Electromagnets produce a changing magnetic field when electric current is passed through them.

For centuries, magnets have been used in an effort to treat pain. There are numerous accounts of shepherds, Greek physicians, and doctors from the Middle Ages using magnets to treat arthritis, gout, and other maladies. The interest in magnets to cure ailments has lasted into the twentieth and twenty-first centuries and has become big business. It is estimated that Americans spend $500 million each year on magnets to treat pain. Worldwide, the estimate leaps to $5 billion spent on magnets.

Fact

Scientific research hasn't concluded that magnets relieve pain despite what the marketing campaigns claim. The FDA also hasn't approved the marketing of magnets that make health claims. In recent years, the FDA and FTC have cracked down on magnet manufacturers and distributors that made health claims.

Theories abound about how magnets might work. These include the idea that static magnets may change cell function, magnets may restore the balance between cell death and growth, and static magnets may increase blood flow and increase oxygen to tissues.

There's also the theory that pulsed electromagnets may alter the brain's perception of pain and electromagnets may affect the production of white blood cells that fight infection and inflammation.

Static magnets are placed on the skin or under clothing so they make contact with the body. Studies of magnets to relieve pain have been too small, not long enough, or lacked a placebo or control group for comparison. There is a need for more rigorous studies of magnets for arthritis-related conditions.

Electromagnets were FDA approved in 1979 to treat bone fractures that had not healed. Researchers have studied the use of electromagnets for knee osteoarthritis and other painful conditions. They haven't been approved for this use and are still considered experimental. If you are going to try magnets, notify your doctor.

L. Essential

In studies that did show some benefit to using magnets, the improvement occurred quickly. The National Center for Complementary and Alternative Medicine suggests buying magnets with a thirty-day money back guarantee and returning them if you don't notice any benefit in one or two weeks.

Bee Stings

Bee stings, bee-venom therapy, and apitherapy are synonymous terminology. Bee-venom therapy is considered an unproven technique, yet there are fifty doctors in the United States that claim their patients have had success treating arthritis with bee therapy.

Bee venom contains eighteen active substances known to have a strong anti-inflammatory effect. One of the substances, mellitin, is said to be 100 times more potent than cortisone. Adolapin, another substance in bee venom, has anti-inflammatory and pain-blocking properties.

Bee-Therapy Research

Bee therapy started after beekeepers noticed that after being stung numerous times, their arthritis symptoms were relieved. The technique is used more commonly in Eastern Europe, Asia, and South America.

One researcher from New Jersey published a study of 108 osteo-arthritis and rheumatoid arthritis patients who had failed conventional treatment. Initially, the study participants received twice-weekly injections. The number of injections was increased until the patients improved. On average, the study participants showed improvement after twelve injections. The study, though, was not a double-blind, placebo-controlled study as is necessary if research is to be taken seriously.

Warning about Bee Therapy

One percent to 5 percent of the population is allergic to bee venom. A patient who is set to start apitherapy or bee therapy must first undergo allergy testing. Though side effects to bee venom are usually mild, people who are allergic to bee stings could have a fatal reaction.

 Alert

Most doctors believe that the risk of an anaphylactic reaction from bee therapy outweighs the unproven benefit of arthritis-symptom relief. There are many treatments to try, alternative and conventional, but they must be safe treatments. Make smart decisions.

Decisions about and preparation for bee therapy should be taken very seriously. Some patients have experienced good results from bee therapy, but have had to stop because the injections or bee stings were too painful. It takes a commitment and it's not easy to endure.

Chapter 10

Exercise Is Vital for Arthritis Patients

THE IMPORTANCE OF EXERCISE for people living with arthritis cannot be overstated. Joint pain and muscle weakness associated with arthritic conditions can be very limiting. You may feel that exercise is secondary to coping with chronic pain, but regular exercise can yield tremendous benefits. Even when results aren't visible or obvious, exercise can lessen the consequences of inactivity. Exercise should be part of a treatment plan tailored specifically for you.

Basic Principles of Exercise for Arthritis Patients

It is a common misconception that people with arthritis cannot exercise because pain associated with the disease is so restrictive. Contrary to this belief, the American College of Rheumatology and the National Institute of Arthritis and Musculoskeletal and Skin Diseases state that regular, appropriate exercise is safe and beneficial for people with arthritis. Exercise:

- Reduces joint pain and stiffness
- Increases flexibility
- Improves muscle strength
- Improves cardiac fitness and endurance

Long-term studies have confirmed that people with inflammatory forms of arthritis (such as rheumatoid arthritis) can participate in moderate-intensity, weight-bearing exercise without increasing pain or disease activity. Less bone loss and joint damage are positive outcomes that can result from exercise for inflammatory arthritis patients. For patients with osteoarthritis, a combination of aerobic and strengthening exercises can improve joint health and function, strength, balance, and coordination.

The key is for exercise to be appropriate for each individual. If you can no longer participate in high-intensity exercise such as athletics, or have to pare back recreational exercise such as distance walking, therapeutic exercise should still have a place in your daily routine. Range-of-motion exercises, strengthening exercises, and aerobic exercises are three types of exercise that are very beneficial for people with arthritis. If you haven't been exercising but you are beginning to realize the importance of it, you may be wondering how to start. Start with your doctor.

Discuss your plan to begin exercising with your doctor. Your doctor can help you decide how to build an exercise regimen designed specifically for you, or you may be referred to a physical therapist or occupational therapist for an evaluation of your physical limitations that will support their recommendations. Once what exercises you should be doing has been determined, start slow and stick with it!

Range-of-Motion Exercises

Range-of-motion exercise, exactly as its name implies, takes each of your joints through their full range of normal movement. On a daily basis, range-of-motion exercises maintain normal movements, help to relieve joint stiffness, and increase flexibility. Range-of-motion exercise consists of gentle, stretching movements and can be done on land or in the water.

The Arthritis Foundation recommends that you should do range-of-motion exercise daily and build up to fifteen minutes per day. When you are able to do fifteen continuous minutes of range-of-motion exercises, you may be able to add some strengthening and aerobic exercises into your routine. Some people find it helpful to do range-of-motion exercises in the morning to quell bothersome morning stiffness.

Strengthening Exercises

People with arthritis must maintain muscle strength by exercising. Strong muscles protect your joints and also support joints weakened by arthritis. Your ability to move depends on your muscle strength.

Isometric and isotonic exercises are two types of strengthening exercises. Isometric exercises tighten the muscles without moving the joint. Isotonic exercises strengthen muscles by moving the joints.

The American College of Rheumatology suggests doing a set of eight to ten exercises (targeting each major muscle group) two to three times a week. Most people with arthritis should perform eight to twelve repetitions of each exercise. Latex or rubber thera-bands, weights, or using a weight machine at a gym can provide resistance. You may find it better to increase the number of repetitions, while decreasing resistance. The Arthritis Foundation recommends that strengthening exercises be done every other day after warming up with range-of-motion exercises.

 Alert

Remember, your exercise routine must be tailored to you. Have a health professional or certified trainer help you construct an exercise program. If you have made up your own routine, have a professional review it to be sure you are on the right course and not risking injury.

Aerobic Exercises

Aerobic exercise is also known as cardiovascular exercise or endurance exercise. Aerobic exercise includes physical activities that use the large muscles of the body in repetitive, rhythmic, and continuous motions. With aerobic exercise, you are working to make your heart, lungs, blood vessels, and muscles work as efficiently as possible. People with arthritis experience side benefits from aerobic exercise, such as weight control, better sleep, less anxiety and depression, and better overall fitness.

Examples of aerobic exercise include walking, aquatic exercise, bicycling, treadmill, and aerobic dance. If done at a moderate pace, everyday activities such as walking the dog, leaf raking, or golfing may be considered aerobic exercise.

The American College of Rheumatology recommends that aerobic exercise consist of thirty to sixty minutes of moderate intensity exercise, three to five days a week. It need not occur in one session, however. The recommended time can be divided into ten-minute segments throughout the day or week.

If your pain level is high, do shorter sessions. Determine your individual tolerance for the exercises planned: If you feel an adjustment should be made to your routine, discuss it with your doctor or the person serving as your exercise advisor. Exercise routines can be adapted and modified, but realize that exercise belongs in your daily routine. You are doing yourself a disservice if you choose to ignore the importance of exercise.

Why Many Arthritis Patients Don't Exercise

Many factors may affect how you think about exercise. Sorting out valid fears from convenient excuses can change a negative attitude toward exercise to a positive attitude. National survey results revealed that 37 percent of people with arthritis get no exercise. Common reasons given for dismissing exercise include:

The pain is too overwhelming—You may feel unable to exercise since it is difficult to stand up. Adaptation is the answer. Many arm exercises can continue unchanged and leg exercises can be modified for a person who is sitting. Pain may be better controlled if exercises are non-weight-bearing or if they are performed in water, where water buoyancy relieves stress and pain around joints.

You think exercise will make arthritis worse—This is a common misconception. Appropriate exercise actually reduces pain, though it may take weeks or months to fully realize the benefit of regular exercise. Be careful not to overwork a joint that is inflamed or painful, while continuing with the rest of your workout. Even if you feel you are in a major arthritis flare, you can still do gentle range-of-motion exercises and add strengthening and aerobic exercises back in once the flare subsides.

You're worried that people will gawk at you—Your concern over your health must take precedence over negative feelings you have about your appearance. Ideally, you should find a supportive group of people to exercise with, such as senior groups or others with arthritis who are looking for support from you the way you are looking for support from them.

A gym membership or the services of a personal trainer can be expensive—Explore all of your options. Consider buying your own inexpensive equipment (such as hand weights) at a discount store and working out in the privacy of your own home. Just remember to have a health professional approve your exercise routine. If you prefer the gym setting, look for local fitness clubs that may be less expensive than well-known gyms. With regard to hiring a personal trainer, try to find one who works with small groups of people and you can split the cost.

The machines at the gym look complicated—Gyms have trained personnel to help instruct you. Ask about machines you are unfamiliar with or other questions you may have. Suffice to say, you will learn! Every person who goes to the gym had a first day at the gym and felt apprehensive.

You are afraid of developing muscles—Unless you plan on participating in an aggressive, competitive bodybuilding campaign, you won't be building unsightly muscles. The goal is not to become muscular, but to strengthen muscles to allow you to remain mobile and able to function independently.

You will give up when results are not quickly apparent—Exercise is not a vehicle for immediate results. If you are looking for immediate results, you will set yourself up to feel discouraged.

Therapeutic exercise is a lifelong process. The goals are long-term, not short-term. Enter into it with patience and a commitment to stick with your exercise plan.

You have no time to exercise—Analyze your daily schedule and look for time when you can exercise. Create a time slot just for that. If that still seems impossible to do, do what you can by walking more, taking stairs more frequently, and consciously being as physically active as you can be while going about your daily routine.

You intend to start another day—Find a reason to start today. Unless you have a temporary, legitimate reason to wait, today is the day. When you are committed to the idea of starting, both physically and emotionally, you have a much better chance of continuing with your exercise regimen and incorporating it into your lifestyle. Why is any other day better than today? Today is the day you start.

Patients may blame their doctor for not recommending exercise as part of their treatment regimen. Other patients think that if their doctor didn't say it, it's not important. Doctors should be involved in prescribing regular exercise, and more exercise programs focused on the needs of arthritis patients should be made available.

Fact

A study in the *Journal of Rheumatology* (September 2003) compared a group of women with osteoarthritis who did Tai Chi for twelve weeks to a group who received standard treatment. The Tai Chi group reported 30 percent less pain and 30 percent improvement in their functional abilities and balance.

As an arthritis patient, you must take responsibility and realize that exercise must be part of your life for your better health. Arthritis doesn't make exercise less necessary; it makes exercise more necessary. Wrap your mind around the importance of exercise and consult your doctor about the best way to approach it.

Tai Chi

If you are interested in a mild or gentle form of exercise, you may have found it with Tai Chi. Practiced for 600 years in China, Tai Chi exercises the mind, body, and spirit. While performing Tai Chi, people move through slow and synchronized positions. Tai Chi postures work the muscles gently, require concentration, and improve the flow of qi (pronounced "chi"), which has been described as "vital life energy that sustains health and calms the mind."

Though Tai Chi originated in China, it has gained popularity in the West. People of all ages can practice Tai Chi. It is especially appealing to people who dislike fast-paced, aggressive exercise.

You can find Tai Chi classes at community centers, karate schools, and possibly HMOs (health maintenance organizations). There are books and videos created to teach Tai Chi, but it is best to have an instructor who can watch you and be sure you are moving properly.

Some doctors recommend Tai Chi to arthritis patients. Tai Chi allows a person to gradually improve flexibility and build muscle strength. The emphasis of Tai Chi is on gentle movement of joints through their range of motion, breathing through the movements, and inner stillness that relieves stress or anxiety.

There are five recognized styles of Tai Chi: Yang (the popular style of today's world), Sun, Wu, Hao, and Chen.

The Arthritis Foundation of Australia and Dr. Paul Lam have developed a program known as Tai Chi for Arthritis. You can learn more on their Web site: *www.taichiforarthritis.com/program.htm*. The program has been adopted by other Arthritis Foundations, including the United States. The program is designed for people without prior knowledge of Tai Chi, relieving pain and stiffness through appropriate forms of

Tai Chi, promoting relaxation, and improving quality of life for people with arthritis.

The program is based on the Sun style of Tai Chi. The Sun style is beneficial for arthritis patients because of steps that enhance mobility, exercises which improve breathing and relaxation, and the use of stances easier for beginners and older persons. There is no bending or squatting with the Sun style of Tai Chi.

Alert

A Tai Chi program is offered by the Arthritis Foundation. The program consists of twelve movements (six basic and six advanced), a warmup, and cool down. (✍www.arthritis.org/events/getinvolved/programsservices/taichi.asp).

Yoga

Yoga is a practice that focuses on the connection between the mind, body, and spirit. The term *yoga* means "to unite" in Sanskrit, the language of ancient India, where yoga originated over 5,000 years ago.

Regular yoga activity can increase muscle strength, improve flexibility, improve respiratory and cardiovascular endurance, improve balance, and reduce pain. It can also relieve stress, anxiety, depression, and insomnia, improve posture and body alignment, and help with weight management.

Many people cringe at the thought of yoga because they associate it with sophisticated pretzel poses that seem impossible to duplicate. Advanced positions are not what you would find in beginner yoga classes, and yoga poses can be modified to your needs and limitations. For that reason, it is important to discuss your interest in yoga with your doctor before signing up for a class. It's imperative to inform your instructor that you have arthritis and specific physical limitations and to share your doctor's advice with your yoga instructor.

According to the American Yoga Association, there are three primary aspects of yoga: exercise, breathing, and meditation. Beyond that, there are over 100 specific types of yoga. Hatha yoga, the type of yoga familiar to most people, focuses on physical movement, posture, and breathing techniques. Classical yoga has eight steps:

- Yama (restraint)
- Niyama (observance)
- Asana (physical exercise)
- Pranayama (breathing technique)
- Pratyahara (preparation for meditation)
- Dharana (concentration)
- Dhyana (meditation)
- Samadhi (absorption or merging of self with the universe)

You can familiarize yourself with yoga from books, Web sites, or videos. It is important to have proper instruction, especially people who have mobility issues or physical limitations. Beginning yoga classes are often offered at community centers, senior centers, the YMCA, or various health and fitness clubs. It's important for you to check the credentials of the yoga instructor—your yoga instructor should be certified. The International Association of Yoga Therapists (IAYT) Web site (*www.iayt.org*) allows you to search for qualified instructors in your area. If you have avoided yoga because you think you are incapable of the required movements, you may be surprised to learn that there are even yoga classes done entirely from the seated position. Chair yoga may or may not be for you, but you must approach yoga by respecting your body and limitations.

Fact

Though yoga has spiritual roots and aims to enhance happiness and enlightenment, there are physical benefits as well. Numerous scientific trials have been published in medical journals deeming yoga a safe, effective way to increase physical activity.

Another variation of yoga is known as viniyoga, which differs from other types of yoga by placing greater emphasis on the link between breath and movement and adaptation of each asana for individual needs. With viniyoga, breath should lead the body into and out of each asana. There is less focus on the form of the asana and more emphasis on the appropriateness of each exercise for the individual.

Remember that a typical yoga class will not necessarily offer the kind of therapeutic yoga a person with arthritis needs. Therapeutic yoga is geared toward giving one-on-one attention to the patient, similar to what you may expect from a physical therapist. It may be wise for you to find a yoga instructor who has experience working with people who have chronic health conditions.

Water Exercise

The warmth of water can be the optimal way to exercise for many arthritis patients. Water provides a gentle and soothing environment. The warmth of the water can increase circulation and the buoyancy of warm water can take pressure off of your joints as you do your exercises. Some people who resist regular types of exercise find that water exercise is actually enjoyable as well as therapeutic.

Talk to your doctor about how to safely exercise in water. Your doctor may want you to have an evaluation by a physical therapist before you participate in water exercise, or you may be referred for supervised pool therapy.

If you are planning on installing a pool or hot tub at your home, part or all of the cost may qualify as a medical expense on your income taxes if your doctor has prescribed the pool/spa as medically necessary. Don't just assume that you do—check with a tax professional to be sure you qualify for the medical deduction.

Heat can relieve muscle aches, reduce joint pain and stiffness, and be relaxing overall. Even with such good benefits, heat is not for everyone. You will also need to consider other health conditions you may have besides arthritis. It bears repeating that you should check with your doctor.

Mild heat rather than extreme heat is recommended for water exercise. In a pool, water temperatures ranging from 83 to 88 degrees Fahrenheit is adequate for exercise. Hot-tub users can usually withstand higher temperatures, but start gradually and allow yourself time to adjust. Don't stay in for a long time initially; build up the time you can safely spend in the hot tub. Most people should not stay longer than ten to fifteen minutes in a hot tub with a temperature range of 98 to 104 degrees Fahrenheit. As an individual, the time or temperature may need to be decreased.

When you first enter the pool, relax in the soothing water before you start your exercises. Begin your exercises gradually once you feel comfortable. Allow a cool-down period after exercising, before you get out of the water.

Essential

The Arthritis Foundation Aquatics Program is a water exercise program designed for people with arthritis and related rheumatic conditions. Classes are usually offered two or three times a week at local indoor pools for 45- to 60-minute sessions. Contact your local Arthritis Foundation office if you are interested in this program.

It is still your responsibility, as with any type of exercise, to know your limitations and not be reckless about pushing your limits. Get the proper guidance so you do not risk injury, and always remain compliant with instructions you are given.

Walking/Cycling

Many people with arthritis can't walk long distances without excruciating pain, but are advised to walk as much as possible because of the health benefits associated with walking. Without question, there are benefits: Walking is considered an endurance exercise and helps to strengthen the heart and lungs; walking improves stamina and lessens fatigue; as a weight-bearing exercise, walking strengthens bones and reduces the risk of osteoporosis; and most importantly, walking strengthens muscles and improves joint flexibility. With inactivity, joints become stiff and muscles become weak. Walking negates some of the bad effects brought on by inactivity.

Fact

Not only are there physical benefits associated with walking, there are psychological benefits. Walking can promote a whole new attitude. You will feel the sense of accomplishment if you participate in a regular walking program, whether it is by yourself or with others.

It can be very discouraging to lose mobility and independence. To realize the benefits of walking and work toward building up your body despite arthritis, is an absolute morale booster. If you want to establish a walking routine, walk around your own neighborhood at first. As you build confidence, choose places to walk which are more interesting. Change your setting so you don't get bored with walking. You should recognize rather quickly that you feel better from regular walking.

Cycling, whether you are using a stationary or free-standing bicycle, is another good way to exercise your joints and muscles gently. Cycling improves strength, balance, and coordination. It is considered a low-impact form of exercise since it doesn't stress the joints. All of the major muscle groups are worked when you are cycling.

You already know how to walk and most likely how to ride a bicycle, so there is no learning that must take place first. You can control the pace and physical demand of your workout. Remember to listen to your pain and make adjustments so you do not risk injury. Make sure your bicycle is comfortable, otherwise you won't stick with it. Set new goals periodically, based on your limitations and your level of improvement. As you extend the distance you are cycling, your sense of achievement will build accordingly. Don't overdo because you feel zealous about your accomplishment. You still have arthritis and have to keep it in perspective. Listen to your pain when you are done with a daily cycling session.

Adjustments must be made to accommodate your physical limitations and to reduce strain while exercising. For example, the bicycle seat height for a person with arthritis should be at a level whereby the leg will not be fully extended while pedaling. The pedal should be set so that the leg is slightly bent when the foot is at the bottom of the pedal stroke.

Inactivity or Sedentary Lifestyles

You have been reading all about the benefits of regular exercise adapted to your physical needs. You can expect improvement in joint flexibility and muscle strength, less fatigue, and better endurance, as well as a better attitude. With a sedentary lifestyle, you get the opposite results. With inactivity, joint flexibility becomes joint stiffness, muscle strength becomes muscle weakness, fatigue is greater and more problematic, and endurance and positive attitude suffer.

Essential

It's a fact that inactivity feeds weakness. You may have a doctor who has not warned you about the negative outcomes associated with lack of exercise. If exercise is important to you, you may do well with a doctor who values the importance of exercise as much as you do.

It's quite easy to fall into a pattern of inactivity. Chronic pain can leave you feeling like you want to do nothing at all. Yet too much bed rest has serious consequences for an arthritis patient. It's somewhat of a vicious cycle—pain leads to bed rest, yet too much bed rest leads to more pain. Ideally, arthritis patients must find the balance between rest and activity. Actually, inactivity is a risk factor for many chronic conditions, not just arthritis.

If you have been progressively becoming more inactive, it will take a conscious effort to change your habits. With the promise of better health overall and better joint health specifically, the decision to change and set healthy goals is awaiting your commitment.

To start, make a list of changes you know you need to make. Make a list of activities you want to begin doing. Decide that regular exercise is part of your life and fit it in. Don't allow yourself to miss your regular exercise session, but if you must miss, don't make it easy. Eliminate something you enjoy doing that day also. Finally, make sure the goals you are setting are realistic.

CHAPTER 11

Diet and Arthritis

THE EFFECT OF DIET ON ARTHRITIS is among the most debated topics with regard to the management or prevention of the disease. The reason for the debate comes from the fact that you will find many more testimonials than scientific conclusions about diet and arthritis. Regimens for eliminating foods thought to worsen arthritis symptoms exist. There are books and Web sites devoted to the subject. With certainty, it can be said that there is no single diet that controls arthritis symptoms for every patient.

Does Elimination Diet Cure Arthritis?

You will find numerous theories about which foods are good to eat and which foods should be avoided by people with arthritis. Some theories point to eliminating whole groups of foods while others focus on pinpointing the specific food that aggravates your arthritis. Rather than an entire food group as the culprit, individual food sensitivities are a more plausible cause for arthritis flares in some people.

It may seem like an overwhelming task to try to find a single food that may cause you to have a nonspecific, allergic-like, immune reaction manifesting itself as joint pain. Elimination diets do exist, but it's an arduous process and some medical experts disregard the process as a fad while others deem it unhealthy.

Nightshade Vegetable Diet

The nightshade diet is probably the most well-known and commonly tried of the elimination diets. The nightshade diet eliminates nightshade vegetables from the diet, which include tomatoes, potatoes, bell peppers, and eggplant. The benefit of eliminating nightshade vegetables is purely anecdotal and nothing has been proven in terms of reducing arthritis symptoms.

Alert

If you want to try an elimination diet, discuss it with your doctor. Plan the period of fasting, what foods will be eliminated, and how you should add foods back into your diet with your doctor's supervision. Be certain you're taking appropriate vitamins to make up for any nutritional loss.

The Dong Diet

The Dong diet is another well-known elimination diet. Red meat, fruits, dairy products, alcohol, additives, and preservatives are all eliminated with the Dong diet. The diet strongly promotes vegetables, with the exception of tomatoes. The Dong diet dates back to a book published in 1980 called *The Arthritic's Cookbook* and another book called *New Hope for the Arthritic* published in 1985, both by Collin H. Dong, M.D. There are no scientific studies that support the Dong diet.

Alkaline Diet

The alkaline diet focuses on eliminating acidic foods such as sugar, coffee, citrus fruits, grains, and nuts for a one-month period. Supporters of the diet point to relief in arthritis symptoms, while opponents of the alkaline diet suggest people either feel better because they lose weight on the diet, and thereby reduce stress on their joints, or because of the placebo effect (the diet works because people expect it to work).

Vegetarian Diet

Vegetarian diets eliminate meat from the diet. There have been some small studies that indicated people with rheumatoid arthritis were helped by a vegetarian diet. Once again, the studies were small and did not reveal significant benefit that would suggest this is a cure or a solution for the majority of people with rheumatoid arthritis.

Fasting and Eating for Health

Dr. Joel Fuhrman is a board-certified physician in private practice in New Jersey, and as a leading expert on nutritional modifications to reverse disease, he has appeared on numerous radio and television programs. He has had vast experience with the nutritional treatment of arthritis and autoimmune diseases and has also had articles published in medical literature. Dr. Fuhrman suggests that dietary modification must be tailored to the individual patient and that a high-nutrient, vegetable-based diet with appropriate supplementation (such as vitamin D and fish oil) is the starting point that can be an effective modality enabling most patients to either reduce or totally avoid the need for medications for rheumatoid arthritis.

Dr. Fuhrman reports that his impressive results in autoimmune illnesses don't hinge solely on the absence of animal products in the diet, but is related to nutrient scoring to assure that an adequate amount of phytochemicals, such as isothiocyanates, are consumed. After enough time on his recommended dietary protocol, rich in green vegetables, Dr. Fuhrman sometimes recommends periodic fasting to be added for patients not receiving adequate results from dietary intervention alone. Fasting (framed by a vegan diet) has been shown to reduce pain and lower inflammatory markers in patients with autoimmune diseases such as rheumatoid arthritis. An extended period of fasting has been shown to result in remission in some patients. More information is available at his Web site (*www .DrFuhrman.com*).

Why Is Weight Important for Arthritis Patients?

The primary reason that weight is important for arthritis patients is a purely physical reason. Carrying less body weight is less stressful on the weight-bearing joints (hips, knees, ankle, back). Extra pounds can increase pain. According to research, as you walk, your hips, knees, and ankles bear three to five times your total body weight. For every pound you are overweight, it is akin to adding three to 5 pounds of extra weight to each knee while you walk. If you lose 10 pounds, that is equivalent to thirty to fifty pounds of stress subtracted from the joint.

Think of what it is like to lift a 10-pound bag of potatoes. That gives you a better idea of how much stress you can relieve from your joints by controlling your weight. Bottom line: Maintaining your ideal body weight is healthy for your joints.

⫶ Essential

Controlling your weight is best done through a regimen that combines dieting by reducing caloric intake with regular physical activity. Cutting 500 calories a day from your total calorie count is a good way to help you lose and keep off weight.

With a loss of 1 to 2 pounds per week, a 10-percent reduction in body weight would take about six months. Gradual weight loss usually keeps extra pounds off rather than quick, fad diets.

Obesity and Osteoarthritis

Being overweight is considered a risk factor for osteoarthritis. Johns Hopkins population-based studies have linked being overweight or obese to developing knee osteoarthritis. One study indicated that women who were obese had four times the risk of developing knee osteoarthritis compared to non-obese women. Obese men had five times the risk of developing knee osteoarthritis.

Weight Management for Better Overall Health

Weight management should be viewed as an integral part of arthritis management. Not only should weight be managed for reasons associated with joint protection, weight loss can help prevent or control other comorbid conditions such as hypertension, heart disease, diabetes, and other health complications.

It takes commitment and a good attitude to make progress toward losing weight. If you aren't ready to commit to a weight loss regimen, then focus on weight maintenance so that you don't gain weight.

Weight Loss Is Not Easy

It's no easy task to lose weight. Since arthritis patients are saddled with the extra burden of chronic pain, it is even more difficult. Keeping your eye on the goal is a big part of strengthening your commitment. First, realize how you will benefit by losing weight. Internalize the reasons for your goal and never lose sight of it. Perhaps writing in a journal will help you keep focused. Finding a support system of one person or many people who are trying to lose weight can help you keep your commitment to your weight loss plan.

According to researchers from Johns Hopkins University School of Medicine in Baltimore, modest weight loss can result in significant improvements in function, stiffness, knee pain, and overall quality of life. In a small study involving forty-eight adults, a weight loss of fifteen pounds triggered a 50-percent improvement in knee pain, stiffness, and function. The fifteen-pound weight loss also correlated with a 40-percent improvement in the ability to do physical tasks, a 20-percent boost in energy, and a 15-percent improvement in the patient's social life.

Healthy, Balanced Diet Is Important

Whether or not you need to lose weight, it's important for people with arthritis to eat a healthy, balanced diet. It's important for everyone to eat a healthy, balanced diet for better overall health. You may have heard the joke, "If I knew I was going to live this long I would have taken better care of myself." Any medical professional will tell you that it's never too late to take better care of yourself.

Diet Advice from Dr. Andrew Weil

Dr. Andrew Weil, a popular health advisor (*www.drweil.com*), recommends an anti-inflammatory diet to people with arthritis, and generally for better long-term health. Dr. Weil recommends these dietary changes:

- Eliminate polyunsaturated vegetable oils and partially hydrogenated oils.
- Eliminate trans-fatty acids.
- Use olive oil instead of vegetable oil.
- Increase your intake of omega-3 fatty acids (salmon, sardines, walnuts, flax seeds or flaxseed oil, soy foods).
- A fish-oil supplement with DHA and EPA can be taken by people who would prefer not to eat fish.
- Eat fresh fruits and vegetables, especially those recognized as high in antioxidants.
- Add ginger and turmeric to your diet.
- Avoid refined and processed foods.

The New Food Pyramid

A new food pyramid was released in 2005 by the United States Department of Agriculture (USDA).

MyPyramid.gov will generate a personalized plan for you. It also explains the types of foods in each food pyramid group, how to count the amounts of food in each group, and other useful tips to promote healthy eating.

Fact

You can find MyPyramid on the Web at *www.MyPyramid.gov*. The new pyramid emphasizes that nutrition and healthy eating is not one-size-fits-all. You can develop your own nutrition plan by entering your age, sex, and level of physical activity in "My Pyramid Plan" at their Web site.

Jumpstarting Better Dietary Habits

It is easy to understand why people with arthritis are less likely to consistently eat a well-balanced, nutritious diet compared to healthy individuals: Chronic pain can interfere with your appetite. Your desire to eat well may rise and fall with your level of pain. Arthritis pain and physical limitations may make meal preparation more difficult. Simply put, you don't feel like eating and you don't feel like cooking.

Some of the medications you take can cause stomach upset or heartburn, steering you away from preparing or eating a nutritious meal. When your pain level is high, comfort foods may seem more appealing, but their nutritional value is likely to be low.

Essential

People with arthritis should have the same goals for good nutrition and good health as any person, perhaps even higher goals. Through various healthy actions, you must stay as healthy as possible in mind, body, and spirit despite having a chronic disease. Eating a healthy, nutritious diet is one of those actions.

A consultation with a registered dietician may be something to consider. A dietician can assess your nutritional needs and evaluate how arthritis is affecting your dietary choices. Sometimes it only takes a bit of guidance to get you back on track. A dietician can make recommendations and create a daily or weekly dietary plan just for you. Your doctor can refer you to a dietician.

Do Certain Foods Cause Arthritis?

Other than individual food allergy or food sensitivity, there has been no causal relationship between food and arthritis proven by large scientific studies or widely accepted. It can be difficult for arthritis patients to sort through testimonials, new research results, and fraudulent diet claims while trying to determine what foods are best to eat and which are best to avoid.

Research Remains Inconclusive

Researchers have been studying the diet-arthritis connection for more than seventy years, but any substantial link has yet to be found. Certain foods have been shown to exacerbate symptoms in some rheumatoid arthritis patients, but their elimination produced short-term results, not long-term results. It was also not possible to distinguish the short-term benefits that were observed from possible spontaneous remission of disease symptoms or from the placebo effect.

In 1990, Dr. Richard Panush published a study in the *Journal of Rheumatology* that is often referred to in discussions about diet and arthritis. Dr. Panush concluded that a small number of rheumatic disease patients (probably not more than 5 percent) have "immunologic sensitivity" to food.

Gout Does Have a Dietary Link

Gout, however, is the exception. Gout, unlike other types of arthritis, has been linked to diet. Gout is caused by excess uric acid in the body. Uric acid is the final by-product of purine metabolism. Purines, which are found in all human tissue, are also found in many foods.

Excess uric acid, also called hyperuricemia, can be caused by an overproduction of uric acid by the body or the underelimination of uric acid by the kidneys. Foods that are high in purines can raise uric acid levels in the blood and cause gout attacks.

Purine-rich foods should be avoided in favor of a diet that includes foods with low to moderate purines. The following foods are considered purine-rich according to the American Medical Association:

- Alcoholic beverages (especially beer)
- Yeast
- Anchovies, sardines in oil, herring, fish roe
- Liver, kidneys, and other organ meat
- Legumes, including dried beans and peas

- Meat extract, including gravy and consommé
- Cauliflower, asparagus, spinach, and mushrooms

Fact

People who have had a gout attack or have chronic gout are advised to avoid a diet that is high in purines. It is not recommended that all purines be eliminated from your diet, since purines are found in all foods which contain protein.

Are There Any Foods You Should Avoid?

Since diet hasn't been tied to the cause of arthritis or the cure for arthritis in any way which would apply to the majority of arthritis sufferers, dietary recommendations are broad.

Arthritis patients should avoid a diet high in fat. They should also limit intake of sugars and salt, alcohol (check with your doctor to see if you are allowed alcohol), and size of food portions. Lupus patients should avoid alfalfa sprouts, since they have been associated with a lupus-like syndrome in monkeys.

Generally, recommendations are for people with or without arthritis and aim to improve general health and maintain ideal weight.

Do Certain Foods Help Arthritis?

Beyond the recommendations for eating a healthy diet, making nutritious choices, controlling food portions, and managing your weight, there are also diets recognized as anti-inflammatory diets.

Is an Anti-Inflammatory Diet Good for You?

Large amounts of arachidonic acid, which you get when you eat animal foods, can increase inflammation. Some arachidonic acid is essential, but too much can worsen inflammation. The American diet consists largely of meat and dairy. The anti-inflammatory diet recommends reducing the amount of saturated fats by decreasing your intake of animal and dairy products.

Alert

There are no diets that offer a miracle cure for arthritis. An anti-inflammatory diet is also not a cure, but the diet recommends substituting foods that produce more inflammatory chemicals with foods that produce less inflammatory chemicals.

Decrease the amount of omega-6 fatty acids, which are found in margarine, corn oil, cottonseed oil, grapeseed oil, peanut oil, safflower oil, sesame oil, soybean oil, sunflower oil, and partially hydrogenated oils. Instead, use monounsaturated oils, such as olive oil or canola oil. Reduce how much filler you eat, such as crackers, pastries, cookies, and chips.

Instead, increase your intake of omega-3 fatty acids, which you will find in cold-water fish (salmon, mackerel, sardines, herring), flaxseeds or flaxseed oil, omega-3 fortified eggs, walnuts, green leafy vegetables, fresh, colorful fruits and vegetables, and by adding ginger or turmeric to your diet.

Eating Better with Gout

The American Medical Association recommends the following dietary guidelines for people with gout, advising them to eat a diet:

- High in complex carbohydrates, such as fiber-rich whole grains, fruits, vegetables
- Low in protein (soy, lean meats, poultry)
- No more than 30 percent of calories derived from fat; 10 percent from animal fats

Recommended foods for gout patients include:

- Fresh cherries, straw-
  berries, blueberries,
  red-blue berries
- Bananas
- Celery
- Tomatoes
- Vegetables, green; leafy
- Pineapple
- Foods high in vitamin C
- 8 glasses of water
  each day

- Fruit juices
- Dairy products
  that are low fat
- Complex carbohydrates
- Chocolate, cocoa, coffee,
  tea, carbonated beverages
- Essential fatty acids
  (tuna, salmon, flax-
  seed, nuts, seeds)
- Tofu may be a good
  alternative to meat

Asparagus, cauliflower, mushrooms, peas, spinach, whole-grain breads and cereals, chicken, duck, ham, turkey, kidney, and lima beans are considered to be moderate in purines and may not negatively affect gout if eaten in reasonable quantities.

To summarize, if you are looking for a diet plan other than the food pyramid recommendations, learn more about the anti-inflammatory diet principles, especially if you have an inflammatory form of arthritis, and the low-purine diet if you have gout.

Vitamins and Arthritis

Vitamins and minerals are important for healthy bodies. According to Johns Hopkins researchers, rheumatoid arthritis patients are commonly observed to suffer deficiencies of the following vitamins and minerals: folic acid, calcium, magnesium, zinc, selenium, vitamins B6 and B12, and vitamins C, D, and E.

Vitamin C

Interestingly, two studies that assessed the role of vitamin C in osteoarthritis and rheumatoid arthritis patients showed different conclusions. Study results that were published in *Arthritis & Rheumatism* (June 2004) indicated that long-term use of vitamin C was associated with increasing severity of knee osteoarthritis. The research was done on guinea pigs. The high doses of vitamin C in guinea pigs produced severe osteoarthritis of the knee and severe cartilage damage. Researchers concluded that vitamin C should not be supplemented above 90 mg/day for men and 75 mg/day for women.

The second study, which was published in the *Annals of Rheumatic Diseases* (2004), reported that foods high in vitamin C protected against inflammatory polyarthritis. In this study, a group of participants who had developed inflammatory polyarthritis over an eight-year period were compared to a group who did not have arthritis. Researchers concluded that the group who had arthritis ate fewer fruits and vegetables than the group without arthritis. Other parameters in the study revealed that the group that consumed the lowest amount of vitamin C was three times more likely to develop inflammatory polyarthritis than those who consumed high amounts of vitamin C.

Dietary Carotenoids

In yet another study, published in the *American Journal of Clinical Nutrition* (August 2005), it was suggested by researchers that some dietary carotenoids may lower the risk of developing arthritis. Beta-cryptoxanthin and zeaxanthin are two of the carotenoids found to lower the risk for developing inflammatory arthritis. Carotenoids are natural pigments found in plants and animals. Beta-cryptoxanthin is a pro-vitamin A carotenoid. It can be converted to the active form of vitamin A in the body. Yellow and orange fruits and vegetables are the best sources of beta-cryptoxanthin.

Folic Acid

Rheumatoid arthritis patients who take methotrexate must take a daily folic acid supplement to prevent side effects associated with folic acid deficiency.

Folic acid is a water-soluble vitamin in the B-complex group. Folic acid, along with vitamin B12 and vitamin C, help with the digestion of proteins and the synthesis of new proteins. Folic acid is needed for red blood-cell production and is also involved in DNA synthesis. Folic acid also plays a role in tissue growth and cellular function.

Eating Well and Vitamin Supplementation

Good health depends on good nutrition. Eating well and making healthy food choices improves overall health, which includes joint health. In this fast-paced world, you may not always eat as nutritiously as you intend. For that reason, most doctors recommend a daily multivitamin to supplement your diet. When you are taking your daily arthritis medications, include a daily multivitamin.

Dietary Supplements

Several dietary supplements have been touted as beneficial for arthritis. Glucosamine-chondroitin (sold in combination or separately), MSM (methylsulfonylmethane), and SAM-e (S-adenosylmethionine) are the most widely known supplements for arthritis. As with any treatment decision you make, you should discuss taking supplements with your doctor. There are many questions associated with dietary supplements for arthritis. Because they are sold over-the-counter, most consumers assume supplements are safe. In reality, they are considered safe for most people, but may be contraindicated in some situations.

Fact

With the exception of vitamin E, taking "natural" vitamins and minerals is no more effective than taking synthetic vitamins and minerals, since natural and synthetic vitamins have equal potency. Synthetic forms of folic acid and vitamin B12 are actually absorbed better than the natural forms.

Glucosamine/Chondroitin

Glucosamine and chondroitin sulfate are both found in normal cartilage. Glucosamine and chondroitin are thought to stimulate the formation of cartilage and play a role in joint repair, but studies have not confirmed their efficacy. Some studies have shown benefit for osteoarthritis pain. Other clinical studies, including the Glucosamine/Chondroitin Arthritis Intervention Trial (GAIT trial), did not conclude that the supplements were effective for osteoarthritis. The supplements are considered safe, though no long-term studies yet exist which confirm long-term safety and effectiveness. Many doctors recommend a trial of glucosamine/chondroitin to osteoarthritis patients for a period of about three months (considered a reasonable time to notice benefit). Patients who are going to try glucosamine/chondroitin are advised to stick with a well-known, reputable manufacturer to assure product integrity.

 Alert

Patients with diabetes should be aware that glucosamine can raise blood-sugar levels. The supplements may also have a blood-thinning effect that may be of concern to patients already taking blood thinners. Glucosamine supplements are derived from shellfish.

MSM (Methylsulfonylmethane)

MSM is a naturally occurring sulfur compound in fresh fruits and vegetables, milk, grains, and fish. Though it is found in foods, as the foods are processed, MSM is destroyed. MSM is also sold as an over-the-counter dietary supplement. It is sold as a solution, tablets, or capsules, and is sometimes sold in combination with glucosamine, chondroitin, or vitamin C. MSM is also sold as a topical cream.

In animal studies involving mice, MSM relieved symptoms similar to rheumatoid arthritis and lupus nephritis. To date, there are two human double-blind, placebo-controlled clinical trials that have indicated MSM is effective for osteoarthritis. The Arthritis Foundation recommends starting with 500 mg twice a day of MSM and increasing gradually to 1,000 mg twice daily, according to the *Arthritis Today* magazine article "MSM-DMSO." Talk with your doctor if you are interested in trying MSM to treat your arthritis symptoms.

Does Drinking Alcohol Affect Arthritis?

It has generally been recommended that adults limit the number of alcoholic drinks to two a day. You, as an arthritis patient, may or may not be able to drink alcohol, depending on what medications you take.

Alcohol and Drug Interactions

There can be serious consequences of mixing certain drugs and alcohol. If you are on methotrexate, you should not be drinking alcohol, unless your doctor allows you a rare special occasion drink. Alcohol can increase the risk of liver toxicity in patients who take methotrexate.

Remember these additional facts about drug and alcohol combinations:

- If you take Tylenol, you should be cautious about drinking alcohol because of the risk of liver damage that may be fatal.
- The combination of alcohol and NSAIDs (nonsteroidal anti-inflammatory drugs) can increase the risk of developing ulcers.
- Analgesic medications (painkillers), muscle relaxants, and sleep medications can intensify the effects of alcohol. Avoid alcohol if you use narcotic analgesics or other central nervous system depressants.

Other Unwanted Problems with Alcohol

Alcohol not only can affect your medications and their effectiveness, it can weaken your bones and pack on unwanted pounds. There are other undesirable consequences of alcohol use for an arthritis patient:

- Chronic and heavy drinking can inhibit the formation of new bone cells, leading to low bone mass.
- Alcohol consumption can induce sleep problems, harmful for arthritis patients already burdened with chronic fatigue.
- Alcohol consumption can increase the risk of gouty arthritis.
- Alcohol increases the permeability of the intestine (e.g., leaky gut syndrome), which some researchers have associated with arthritis.

Alcohol: Not a Coping Mechanism

Though you may look to alcohol as a way of coping with the difficulties of living with arthritis or to make you forget your problems, alcohol can add to your problems. If you have an accident or slip or fall, your arthritis would become more painful from your injuries. When you have arthritis, you must take care of yourself more than ever before, and alcohol does not fit into your plans.

If you are looking to alcohol for help, it may be a sign of depression. Consider seeking treatment for depression or anxiety associated with chronic arthritis.

You shouldn't let alcohol stop you from eating well, exercising, sleeping well, or being compliant with your treatment plan. It is best to avoid alcohol, except for the occasional drink your doctor may allow you on special occasions.

Think about why you are drinking. Are you drinking to diminish your pain? Are you drinking because you feel overwhelmed? Are you drinking because you are angry, frustrated, depressed, or feel hopeless? If the answer is yes, consider consulting with a psychologist who specializes in helping people who live with chronic disease.

CHAPTER 12

Joint Protection

ACTIVITY CAUSES YOU to move your joints. Whether the activities are work related, recreational, or daily living tasks, adhering to joint protection principles and concentrating on good body mechanics will help you avoid exacerbation of arthritis symptoms. Something as simple as learning how to pick up a box properly can protect your joints from further damage.

Recognize the difference between proper and improper movements so that moving in a way that is less stressful becomes second nature. Unnatural stress on a joint can do harm.

Principles of Joint Protection

There are specific techniques and principles that will help you protect your joints. Here are a dozen tips to help you protect your joints: Don't disregard pain; recognize it as a signal to stop what you are doing. Consciously notice when pain and fatigue interrupt activities and take breaks as needed. Pace yourself, especially when activities are more strenuous. Move every joint gently through its full range of motion every day—preserving range of motion is an important aspect of joint protection. Strengthen your muscles by exercising regularly—strong muscles help protect joints. A physical therapist can teach you which exercises will benefit you the most. Be aware of the position of your hands when using them, and avoid stress and strain on your fingers. Use the largest and strongest joint possible for a specific task. For example, carry a tote bag over your shoulder rather than carrying it with your fingers or by looping it over your elbow.

Avoid positions or motions that contribute to ulnar drift or ulnar deviation. Examples include twisting a jar lid in the direction of your little finger or wringing out a dish towel. Motion should be toward the thumb whenever possible. Avoid clenching your fist and straining finger joints and knuckles. Avoid holding objects between your thumb and fingers. For example, when reading a magazine, put it on your lap or support it with your palms.

Don't stay in one position for long periods of time; moving around will decrease stiffness. If you will be driving a long distance, stop and stretch every hour. Don't carry heavy items—use carts to transport heavy items or a load of items. When traveling, your luggage should have wheels. Most importantly, do not start an activity which you would be unable to stop if pain suddenly developed (e.g., traveling on a long road trip and being unable to reach your destination). Pain which persists for two hours after an activity indicates the activity was too stressful for your body.

One of the most obvious ways to protect your joints is to maintain your ideal body weight. Carrying additional body weight adds more stress to your joints, especially the weight-bearing joints (hips, knees, ankles, feet, and back). Reduce the risk of joint damage by shedding extra pounds.

Use common sense. If a prior activity caused joint pain, don't repeat the activity without making adjustments to reduce the stress and strain on your joints. Don't move suddenly without thinking about your movements. Be aware of how you should be moving and how you are moving.

Joint damage and joint deformity can impede normal function. It may become more difficult to do your job, cook and clean, keep up with housework, and maintain personal hygiene. Any activity that involves using damaged joints may be greatly impacted. Manual dexterity and mobility may be severely reduced depending on the degree of joint damage.

Joint protection measures will help preserve function. Your ability to function, in turn, will preserve your independence.

Alert

Delegate! Give the chore that has become a virtual impossibility for you to someone else. Asking for help is not a sign of weakness. Don't risk injury by trying to do things you can no longer do. Don't do without because you cringe at the notion of needing help and view it as a sign of losing your independence.

Body Mechanics

Body mechanics essentially refers to the position of your body when you're moving. Proper body mechanics are important for every person, not just those with arthritis or other musculoskeletal conditions. Correct body position, which is important at all times, can help alleviate pain, reduce stress on your joints, and reduce the risk of injury.

Think about what you do in a typical day. As you stand, sit, walk, drive, lift, reach, and sleep, be aware of your body position. Improving your posture during each phase of activity or rest will help you protect your joints. Proper posture:

- Correctly aligns bones and joints
- Decreases wear and tear on joints
- Reduces stress on ligaments which support the bones in a joint
- Keeps the spine healthy
- Strengthens muscles and conserves energy
- Prevents stress and strain on joints
- Prevents muscle pain

Proper posture requires good muscle tone, normal movement of the joints, and balanced muscle on the sides of the spine.

Optimal Standing Position

Hold your head straight (your earlobes should be above the mid-shoulder point). Good posture while standing consists of shoulder blades back, chest forward, knees straight, and the top of your head aiming for the ceiling. Your pelvis should not tilt. Arches of your feet should be supported with shoes.

Essential

Pain associated with arthritis can increase muscle tension. Poor body mechanics also can increase muscle tension. Muscles that are weak or tense can contribute to pain and improper body mechanics. It's a cycle you have to break by managing pain and strengthening muscles.

Optimal Sitting Position

When sitting in a chair, your buttocks should be all the way to the back of the chair. Your back should be straight and your shoulders should be back. Some chairs have lumbar features to help support your back. Knees, bent at right angles, should be at the same height or higher than your hips. Feet should be flat on the floor. Avoid crossing your legs.

Optimal Driving Position

When driving, move your seat forward until you feel you are in a comfortable position. Your knees should be slightly bent, and your foot should reach the gas pedal and brake easily. Your knees should be at the same height or higher than your hips. Lumbar cushions offer additional back support.

Optimal Walking Position

A proper gait that incorporates good posture and good body mechanics will help conserve energy as you walk. Strong muscles improve your gait. Arthritis patients who have severely damaged joints or who have had joint surgery may have an abnormal gait. A less-than-perfect gait does not mean you cannot benefit from walking. Orthopedic surgeons advise people to walk as far as they can and as often as they can. Walking builds muscle strength that in turn helps to protect joints.

Optimal Lifting Position

Avoid lifting heavy boxes or objects. If you must lift, plant your feet firmly on the ground and spread them slightly apart for balance. Bend at your knees and hips and lower your body down to meet the object you are trying to pick up. Never bend at the waist while keeping your legs straight and reaching down to grasp the object. As you rise, keep the object close to you.

Optimal Sleeping Position

Whether you sleep on your side, back, or stomach, you should have one pillow underneath your head. Don't rest your shoulders on the pillow—that's a common mistake. Only your head should be on the pillow to allow for proper alignment.

People who sleep on their back may be helped by using a pillow under the knees or a lumbar roll under the lower back. Those who sleep on their side should sleep with knees slightly bent. The position required for sleeping on the stomach isn't actually optimal for your neck or back.

The firmness of your mattress should be comfortable while still offering good support. A good night's sleep on a supportive mattress can reduce pain and protect your joints.

Using Assistive Equipment/Assistive Devices

Damaged joints can make it difficult to perform the usual tasks of daily living. Painful joints, weak muscles, limited range of motion, and joint deformity can make the simplest of tasks a challenge for people with arthritis. You have to adjust and adapt to your physical limitations. A variety of assistive/adaptive equipment is available to help you make necessary adjustments and protect your joints as well. Adaptive equipment is designed to reduce stress and strain on your joints. Determine what tasks you need help with and what is most problematic for you. Make a list and then begin to problem solve.

Housecleaning

Many people who are not limited by arthritis view housecleaning as drudgery. If you can't easily reach, bend, or scrub, it's even worse drudgery. There are myriad ergonomic cleaning tools available. Long-handled mops, long-handled shower scrubbers, long-handled ceiling fan dusters, and long-handled light bulb changers help compensate for limited range of motion. Self-propelled vacuum cleaners help preserve energy. Cleaning tools that are easy to grip and have extended handles are not only more convenient, they are less strenuous on your joints.

If you are still unable to complete certain tasks after trying various assistive devices, you may need to look for outside help, such as a housekeeper or handyman. First, try to get referrals from people you know. If that turns out to be a dead end, check out Angie's List at *www.angieslist.com.*

Kitchen Work

Look for kitchen equipment that is easy for you to use. There are hands-free can openers, automatic jar openers, electric potato peelers, and stand mixers available. You also need baking pans with secure handles and a set of nonstick cookware. Make sure your dishes are lightweight.

Organize your kitchen shelves to suit your needs. Frequently used items shouldn't be stored in hard-to-reach places. Everything in your kitchen should be convenient and easily accessible.

Prepare extra when you cook so you will have leftovers or meals you can freeze for a later time. On days you don't feel like cooking, you will appreciate a good meal waiting for you in the freezer.

Grocery Shopping

Tackling a long grocery list may feel like a workout. Besides a lot of walking, it takes some endurance to load items into the cart, unload at the cash register, load into your car, and unload again at home. Consider your alternatives. Smaller but more frequent shopping trips may be one solution.

Another alternative is to check and see if your area has grocery delivery available. Some larger grocery chains offer online shopping, where you select your groceries and the time and day you want it delivered. If this is available to you, give it a try!

Laundry

Rolling laundry carts eliminate the stress and strain of lifting heavy laundry baskets. Smaller, more manageable loads may be an adaptation you need to consider also. Long-handled reacher aids can help you reach the back or bottom of your washer and dryer. Setting up a table near your washer and dryer can help with laundry sorting or folding.

Driving

From small items to major modifications, cars and vans can be adapted to your needs. Specially designed key fobs for people with disabilities allow a better grip and more stability when turning the key to start the ignition. Gas cap wrenches are available which add leverage needed to open the gas cap easily. If getting into or out of the car is a problem for you, a six-way power seat is an option on some vehicles (adjusts the seat up and down, adjusts the angle of the back of the seat, and the seat moves closer to or farther from the steering wheel). Some car manufacturers may offer rebates to help modify your car to make it more accessible or install more power features.

There are many catalogs available online which offer assistive devices and adaptive equipment. Not only gadgets, but supports and mobility equipment such as canes, crutches, wheelchairs, and scooters are available. Search Google for "arthritis aids catalogs."

Pain Management

It may take many attempts, but finding the best way to manage your pain is a priority. As a way of alerting you that something is wrong, acute pain is a good thing. Chronic pain, though, is purely an intruder in your life.

Pain physically impacts your body by tensing muscles, limiting mobility, contributing to fatigue, and robbing you of energy. Pain also has an emotional impact and it can be the catalyst for anger, depression, and fear.

 Fact

Arthritis is strongly associated with major depression, likely because of functional limitations imposed by the disease, according to the Centers for Disease Control and Prevention (CDC). Up from 16 million in 2002, now 17.4 million American adults with doctor-diagnosed arthritis report arthritis-attributable activity limitations.

Living better with arthritis and managing your pain are synchronous goals. The physical and emotional impact of uncontrolled pain can interfere with every aspect of your life. The goal of pain management is to diminish pain as much as possible and improve your quality of life.

People experience and react differently to pain. Tolerance of pain varies between different individuals. Various nerves are involved in receiving and transmitting pain signals. When a pain signal is sent, the body releases chemicals to try to block the pain signal. In chronic pain situations, pain continues even when pain stimuli (e.g., inflammation) are controlled. You must have a pain management plan tailored to your specific condition.

In most cases, medications will play a significant role in pain management. Other pain management options may include: injections (i.e., corticosteroid or epidural), physical or occupational therapy, acupuncture, acupressure, relaxation techniques, massage, chiropractic, TENS or electrical stimulation, and joint surgery.

If your pain is well-managed, you will be able to focus on other actions that will help you protect your joints from further damage and deformity (good posture, exercise, staying active). Pain can exaggerate already poor body mechanics. You may slouch or walk hunched over. You may take smaller steps when walking, or favor one side more than the other. Muscle atrophy and joint deformity can result. With effective pain management, bad habits that contribute to making pain worse can be corrected.

Consult your rheumatologist and discuss your options. You should also consider consulting with a pain medicine specialist. A physical therapist or occupational therapist may also become part of your pain-management team.

Don't be alarmed if you feel frustrated while you are trying to effectively manage your pain. Be prepared for pain to flare up at unexpected times. Even with treatment, many factors will affect your pain level. Besides the aforementioned pain management options, there are positive attributes that will help you manage your pain. Positive attitude, perseverance, and courage will guide you to make right choices that will help you manage your pain. Pain management requires a multidisciplinary approach. A combination of effective treatments and positive actions has a greater chance of successfully managing pain than any single treatment option.

Preserving Range of Motion

The extent of normal movement for a joint caused by flexion (bending), extension (straightening), abduction (away from midline), adduction (toward the midline), and rotation is referred to as range of motion.

An understanding of how the synovial joints move will help you realize how important it is to protect your joints. The end of the two bones that come together to form a synovial joint are covered by a slippery surface known as articular cartilage. The cartilage serves as a cushion to absorb shock, and also allows for unimpeded movement of the bones. The synovial joint is encapsulated and has a synovial lining within the joint capsule. Within the joint, there is a relatively small amount of synovial fluid which lubricates the joint.

The most common synovial joints include:

- Ball-and-socket joints (hip, shoulder)
- Ellipsoidal joints (joint at base of index finger)
- Gliding joints (some bones in ankles and wrists)
- Hinge joints (knee, elbow)
- Pivot joint (in neck, allows head to move from side to side)
- Saddle joint (in thumbs)

Joints that are painful may need to be stabilized or splinted to allow rest and reduce stress. You don't want to continue to stress any joint which is already painful. Continuously using a splint or support is not good, however. It's best for you to exercise the painful joint gently, taking it through its full range of motion. As the joint becomes less painful, you should add activities so the joint is used, rebuilding muscle tone and function.

Essential

There are three classifications of joints according to Henry Gray's *Anatomy of the Human Body:* synarthroses (immovable), amphiarthroses (slightly moveable), and diarthroses (freely movable). Most joints in your body are diarthrodial joints, more commonly referred to as synovial joints.

Daily, gentle exercise which takes a joint through its range of motion is optimal, rather than a sporadic exercise schedule. Range-of-motion exercises will help you maintain joint flexibility.

Exercises for your neck

- Gently turn your head to the right, return to the front, and then turn to the left.
- Tilt your head to one shoulder and then to the other shoulder.

Exercises for your fingers and knuckles

- Close your hand, then open it.
- Touch thumb to each fingertip, one at a time.
- Spread fingers wide apart, then bring back together.

Exercises for your legs, knees, hips

- Sit straight in a chair. Lift knee straight up about 3 inches off of the chair. Repeat with other knee.
- Sit in a chair in normal position. Straighten leg out at the knee, then bring knee back down and have foot rest on the floor. Repeat with other leg.
- Lying in bed, do leg raises by moving at the hip and keeping knee straight. Repeat with other leg.
- Lying in bed, move leg out to the left and bring it back to center. Repeat with other leg.
- Stand facing a wall. Balance yourself by placing your hands on the wall. Lift leg backwards. Repeat with other leg.

Exercises for ankle motion

- Bend foot down at the ankle, then bend foot up.
- Make circular motions with your ankles, one at a time.

Exercises for elbows

- Straighten your arm at the elbow in front of you. Then bend arm up again at the elbow.
- Straighten arm at elbow, then return your arm to bent position. Then raise your arm up toward the ceiling.

Exercises for shoulders
- Lying down, raise arm at the shoulder above your head, keeping elbow straight.
- Stretch arm across body as far as it will go.
- Reach one arm up and try to pat yourself on the back. Reach the opposite arm behind your lower back. Try to touch your hands. Switch arms and repeat.

Exercises for wrists
- Curl wrist in and then move it back out.
- Make circular motions with your wrists.

Exercises for lower back
- Bend at the waist.
- With arms on your hips, bend to the right, come back to center, then bend to the left.

A physical therapist can show you a beginning exercise regimen and work with you to build upon your regimen. The physical therapy consult assures you are doing exercises properly and in good form.

Fact

According to the U.S. Department of Labor, physical therapists encourage patients to use their own muscles to increase their flexibility and range of motion before finally advancing to other exercises that improve strength, balance, coordination, and endurance. The goal is to improve how an individual functions at work and at home.

Avoiding Stress and Strain on Joints
You've read about how joint protection principles, proper body mechanics, assistive devices, and pain management are all necessary

for you to be able to reduce stress and strain on your joints. Keep the following tips in mind as well.

Supports and braces can add stability to joints. A stable joint is less likely to become damaged or injured. You should not continue to walk on an unstable, unsupported joint. Instability can cause injury or lead to joint damage.

Your joints are more easily strained if they are already swollen, warm, inflamed, and painful. Be extra cautious with your joints when they are already hurting. Take steps to treat the symptoms and reduce your activity level until symptoms are better controlled.

Wait twenty-four hours to resume normal activities after receiving a joint injection, otherwise you risk straining the joint involved. Don't use joint injections to mask pain in an effort to accelerate activity. There is a risk of joint damage by using joint injections for that reason.

Don't ever increase your pain medications beyond their maximum daily allowable dose. There is a limit on how much pain medication you can safely take. If you are unsure, ask your doctor.

When doing range-of-motion exercises, active range of motion means you need no assistance. You can do passive range of motion also, where you assist yourself (e.g., one of your arms helps to lift the other) or another person assists you. Either way, you're putting your joints through their full range of motion, which is your daily goal.

If you feel you have strained a joint, use R.I.C.E. (Rest, Ice, Compression, and Elevation) to help you recover. Inability to bear weight on your foot, ankle, or leg indicates you may have a severe strain. Seek medical attention or medical advice.

Repetitive motion can cause stress and injury to muscles, joints, and tendons. Remember to vary your position as much as possible. To help reduce stress from repetitive motion, dangle your arms and then put your hands behind your head and arch your back. While standing, with your hands on your hips, lean backwards to arch your back.

Remember to create a workstation or work environment that emphasizes ergonomics. If you spend much of your day at work or working at home, you must be sure that your setup is not contributing to joint pain and joint damage.

Pain, disease, and joint damage are the most frequent causes of limited range of motion. To preserve your range of motion you need to control pain, treat the disease, and reduce the risk of joint damage. Rest when you need to, but don't become sedentary. Mobility helps decrease joint stiffness. Be as active as possible, but don't overdo to the point of straining your joints; find the balance.

Make adjustments as necessary to improve joint health. Some adjustments may be minor and others may be major. You don't want to have to stop working or give up activities. To preserve your ability to work and to be active, you must preserve your joints. Pay close attention to how your joints feel and to any changes you begin to feel in your joints. Don't ignore subtle changes—let your doctor decide if it's anything that requires medical attention.

Joint health directly correlates with mobility and function. Declining joint health pushes you toward disability. It is easier to protect your joints and maintain good function than to lose function and have to try to regain it.

CHAPTER 13

Arthritis Brings a New Reality

IT'S MUCH EASIER TO TALK about the basic facts of arthritis than to consider the uncertainties of living with a chronic disease. On a day-to-day basis, aspects of what are considered "normal living" can be affected by arthritis. Your home life and work life can be changed. As you would expect, people with disabling types of arthritis and those with a severe course of the disease face the most change in their lives. In most cases, the new reality arthritis brings occurs gradually.

Can You Keep Working?

As arthritis progresses, depending on your job responsibilities, it may become increasingly difficult to continue working. People who have physical jobs and spend a majority of the work day standing, walking, lifting, or reaching, as well as people whose jobs require manual dexterity, face challenges which may become greater if arthritis is uncontrolled or symptoms worsen.

It's hard to know what to do as working becomes more difficult. It becomes a tug of war between hanging on to your job and acknowledging you can no longer work. It's probably one of the most difficult decisions you will ever have to make—deciding that you are truly disabled and can no longer work. Many people faced with that decision feel that the disease has won if they concede to being disabled. It should not be viewed as winning or losing; arthritis can be life changing and it brings new realities.

Twenty years ago, over one half of individuals with rheumatoid arthritis who worked before onset of the disease stopped working within ten years of diagnosis. It is one of the goals of newer treatments to keep people working longer and prevent disability. Clearly, people with arthritis try to work as long as possible, both for economic reasons and for the satisfaction that comes from living a productive life. Being aware of how arthritis can affect your ability to work may help you plan ahead and make adjustments that will keep you working.

 Fact

According to the CDC, arthritis and other rheumatic conditions are recognized as the leading cause of disability in the United States. Approximately 30.6 percent of adults aged 18–64 with doctor-diagnosed arthritis report an arthritis-attributable work limitation.

Communicate with Your Employer

It's a common dilemma for people who are having difficulty at work—should you tell your boss arthritis is affecting your work or should you hide it as long as you can? The fear of losing your job may hold you back from talking to your boss and opening up the lines of communication. It's up to you to decide when the time is right to discuss your medical condition with your boss or employer. Don't assume the discussion will have a negative impact on your job, though. With the right approach, you may be able to find a solution that will help you stay on the job and perform better.

Depending on your work responsibilities, you may be able to request a flexible schedule, adaptations to your work environment, a different position that is less physically demanding, and a change from full time to part time.

Be aware that some of the changes listed above may result in alterations to your benefits. Before you change positions or switch from full time to part time, discuss the effect it may have with your employer or benefits manager. The change may keep you working and may be worth a cut in pay or less benefits if it comes to that. You want to make informed decisions and avoid surprises.

Communicate with Your Co-workers

You may find solace in the understanding you will receive from your co-workers. Be open with them and help them understand. Explain why certain tasks are difficult for you or why you limp some days but not others. Don't expect them to know and don't be annoyed at their lack of knowledge with regard to arthritis.

You still have a responsibility to be productive at your job. No one is going to do your job for you. Yet, the small acts of kindness your co-workers may offer from time to time, such as lifting a box for you or reaching something from a top shelf, can help tremendously. Even just having their moral support throughout the workday is uplifting.

Knowing When It's Time to Stop Working

How do you know when it's time to stop working? If you're still asking yourself that question, it's not the right time. Many doctors advise that you should keep working for as long as you can. When your work is negatively impacting your quality of life, then you should seriously consider applying for disability. Prepare for the day you have to quit your job, with the hope that it may never come. Preparedness will allow you to make the right decision at the right time.

Can You Have a Baby?

Many women develop arthritis during their childbearing years. There are many factors that go into the decision to have a baby for women without health problems, but there are even more for those who have health concerns. The decision should be made after discussing your plans with your rheumatologist. There is no clear-cut answer to whether you can or should have a baby if you have chronic arthritis. It depends on the individual woman, the severity of disease, and the level of disability, as well as the medications that you may be required to take for your arthritis during a potential pregnancy.

Considerations Before You Become Pregnant

Women who are planning to become pregnant must discontinue certain medications, especially immunosuppressants. With the recommendations of your doctor, you must decide if your arthritis is stable enough so that you can stop medications. You must formulate a plan for how you will deal with flaring of arthritis symptoms that may occur. You must decide, along with your doctor, if you are physically strong enough in your weight-bearing joints to withstand the additional weight that comes with pregnancy.

☐, Essential

Many women with rheumatoid arthritis experience a remission that often occurs by the end of the fourth month of pregnancy. Attributed to hormonal changes, the remission does not continue after pregnancy is over. It is common for a flare of symptoms to occur two to eight weeks after giving birth.

Ultimately, you must consider how pregnancy will affect your arthritis and vice versa. If you decide you are able to become pregnant, and that any physical discomfort that may result is worth the blessing of being able to have a child, follow the guidance of your doctors.

Most women with arthritis can have a normal course of pregnancy. Depending on what joints are involved, you may require a Cesarean section, though. If you decide you can't have a baby, feel no shame. It may be sad to come to that realization, but once again, arthritis brings new realities to your life. Adoption may be a possibility to fulfill your new reality, but this is a very personal decision.

Taking Care of Baby

The pregnancy itself is just one issue. After you give birth, there is an infant who is totally dependent on you. To test your readiness and your stamina, use a 10-pound bag of potatoes or a similar bundle of the approximate weight of a newborn baby. Practice your ability to lift the bundle, walk up and down stairs with it, and cradle it in your arms for a period of time. Literally go through the motions of bathing, feeding, changing, and dressing the baby.

Anticipating any problems you may have is important. You may need a little help with certain baby-care tasks. Is there someone available to help you? You may need to buy equipment or adapt equipment to suit your needs. Think of what you will need and prepare ahead of time.

Will Arthritis Affect My Baby?

Many parents-to-be wonder if their child will inherit arthritis. If the answer was definitive, it might become part of the decision-making process. There is no definitive answer to the question, though. Scientists have associated certain genetic markers with certain types of arthritis, but the connection between the genetic markers and child development is unclear. It cannot be concluded that your child will develop arthritis because you have genetic markers for arthritis. Even if it can be said that heredity is a factor, it is only one factor and there are others.

Statistically speaking, women with rheumatoid arthritis have a greater likelihood of premature births and newborn complications. There is also a higher risk of miscarriage. With types of arthritis which have systemic complications (lupus, scleroderma), there can be life-threatening complications if the mother already has kidney problems, hypertension, or lung problems. High-risk pregnancy must be closely followed by your rheumatologist as well as your OB-GYN doctor.

Can You Raise Your Kids?

It is definitely possible to be a good parent and have arthritis. First and foremost, the best thing you can do for yourself and your children is to do all that you can do to improve your own health. Approach your health situation positively and effectively and do the same with parenting.

You will learn many lessons while living with chronic arthritis—lessons about the disease and lessons about life. When your children are old enough to understand, explain why Mom or Dad is sick some of the time in terms they can comprehend. Encourage questions and don't be afraid to answer honestly. The more comfortable your children can become with your new reality, the less they will focus on unrealistic fears (e.g., that you're going to die soon). Just as you relaxed the more you learned about arthritis, your kids should be given the same opportunity to learn.

Being the Parent You Envisioned

As a parent, you may feel inclined to make up for being sick by pushing beyond your physical limitations. You may neglect your own health and fail to conserve needed energy.

It's often said that quality time is what counts between a parent and child; it's the time spent together that matters. If you can no longer throw a football with your son or sew doll clothes for your daughter, think of all the things you can still do. Start by eating dinner together every night. Then think of other activities that bring you and your child together but are not physically draining for you such as watching TV or movies together, taking the dog for short walks together, and working on puzzles or playing board games.

Question

How can I keep pace with my children like I did before I was diagnosed with arthritis?
Don't try to do what you no longer can do at the expense of your health. If your children observe that you are adjusting and adapting to the reality of your physical condition, they will naturally adjust and adapt as well.

Finding the Balance

You must find the balance between family time and time you need for yourself. Your parenting skills will suffer unless you take the time needed just for you. Whether the time is spent going to doctor appointments, going to exercise class, going for a massage, or getting your hair done, that time is for you to improve your health or just relax and destress. Consider spending equal amounts of time on your family and on yourself. That balance may work to keep you from feeling overwhelmed by having a chronic disease, a job, and a family, all of which need your attention.

Adjust the time spent on each so that you feel none of your responsibilities is neglected and you are not neglecting yourself, either. You can do it if you set your priorities and remember you are one of those priorities.

Does Your Social Life Implode?

You may not feel like socializing when pain and other arthritis symptoms are especially bothersome. There is no minimizing the impact arthritis can have on your social life. You may have to consciously put yourself into social situations to ensure your social life does not become extinct. Recognize the problems that you have and try to find solutions.

Going to the Movies or a Concert

Seating may be a problem if you have hip or knee arthritis. It may be difficult to get up from low seats: Don't let that keep you away. Perhaps it would help to bring a pillow or cushion to raise you up. If you are going to a movie, some of the seats are close to railings and that may help you get up more easily. Sit closer to the front so you can forgo the stairs. Don't be shy about admitting you need a little extra consideration from friends or family members who are going with you.

Be sure you get the seats you need (e.g., handicapped seats or seats at the end of a row). If you don't take the time to check, you may end up in seats which are uncomfortable or inaccessible and the experience will be ruined.

Walk 'Til You Drop

There are many situations that require a lot of walking. You may be inclined to avoid such situations—it may seem easier to just skip it. The problem with skipping it is that it compounds feelings that you are missing out. The negative feelings associated with that can increase stress and depression, which in turn exacerbates pain.

You may be thinking you have no control; you just can't walk far. Perhaps that's so—unassisted. Try using assistive equipment such as canes, walkers, wheelchairs, or electric scooters. You may get much farther if you do and you may not have to miss out after all.

⌐ Essential

At concerts or other live performances, plan ahead. Don't just purchase any seat without knowing whether it's suitable for you. Talk to someone in the box office, either in person or on the phone, and discuss your special needs. You will find that the majority of venues are very accommodating.

Party Pooper?

Many people with chronic arthritis, mobility problems, or high levels of pain are turned off by the thought of attending a large party, especially ones that will be attended by acquaintances rather than close family and friends. You may think it's not worth your effort. You never enjoy yourself and it's better to stay home, right?

It's hard to put on a happy face when you're in pain. You can't stand for a long period of time. You don't know where you will be able to sit. You don't drink, and shaking hands hurts! You can give in to all of that; they are all legitimate concerns. You can also look for real solutions and not feed your inclination to isolate yourself. For example, call your host or hostess and ask if they would mind making sure there will be a firm seat available. If someone sits in your seat and you need to sit, politely explain your situation. People are very accommodating when they understand.

If you don't drink and want to avoid having to repeat that over and over throughout the evening, keep a half full glass in your hand

and take sips. To avoid the pain of shaking hands (literally), keep that drink in your right hand. Become creative with your solutions. Don't convince yourself you don't belong at the party.

When You Have to Cancel

Even when you have the best of intentions and try to remain socially active, arthritis will still force you to cancel a date or an event from time to time. Don't make canceling easy, even when necessary. If it becomes easy to cancel, you may begin to develop a pattern. To avoid the trap of isolation, be sure that you reschedule every date or event which must be cancelled.

Does Sex Become a Distant Memory?

As with any activity, intimate or otherwise, pain and fatigue associated with arthritis can interfere with desire. Limited range of motion and physical deformities can also contribute to problems with the mechanics of a sexual relationship. Then, there are emotions that can get spun around. Hopefully, a healthy sexual relationship between committed partners does not become a distant memory. Without question, arthritis can make it more difficult.

Nurturing desire and emotions can improve intimacy. It will require attention from you and your partner, and a conscious effort to not let arthritis destroy a significant aspect of your relationship. Start with good communication.

Communication

It's more important than ever that you communicate your thoughts and needs to your partner. You can't expect your partner to know how you are feeling without open and honest communication. It's both your responsibility and your partner's responsibility to keep an open exchange of thoughts and feelings and to refrain from shutting down when things get difficult.

Fact

> Chronic illness can cause serious difficulties between partners. Some problems can be complex and unresolvable. According to Chris McGonigle, Ph.D., author of *Surviving Your Spouse's Chronic Illness: A Compassionate Guide,* statistics indicate that about 85 percent of marriages faced with challenges caused by one partner being chronically sick eventually fail.

It's not uncommon in intimate relationships for the partner who has arthritis to lose interest in a physical relationship when pain becomes all-consuming. With the hope that tomorrow will be a better day, a pattern can develop if you don't consciously knock down walls you begin to build around yourself. Talk to your partner openly. Let your partner know how to help you.

It's also not uncommon in intimate relationships for the partner who doesn't have arthritis to silently suffer feelings of rejection. A pattern may develop where you appear disinterested, though you are actually unable to overcome pain and fatigue. If you're not communicating, you can send wrong signals.

Change What You're Doing

If your relationship with your partner is suffering, change what you're doing. Not unlike any of the aforementioned activities, you have to make a conscious effort to stay involved. This is even more important because you're talking about the most important relationship in your life.

If pain and fatigue are the factors interfering most in a healthy sexual relationship, make sure you are doing all you can do to manage your disease. Not only should you be open with your partner, you can discuss problems you are having with your doctor. Tap into your doctor's expertise for ideas that will make a difference. Perhaps it would help to take medications at a different time or to add a new medication to better control pain. Gentle exercise or a warm shower before bedtime may be soothing, relaxing, and mood-setting.

From Athlete to Spectator?

If you were an athletic person who enjoyed participating in competitive sports prior to the onset of arthritis, you may be facing a new reality as well. Depending on your individual condition, and your ability to run, jump, throw, and participate in sports aggressively, you may have to make some changes. Your body lets you know what you're no longer able to do. Pain is a signal that something is wrong; if you're having a lot of pain after a sports activity, you must listen to your body.

Consider Acceptable Alternatives

It may be the case that you can no longer participate in a specific sport, but are there others that are not quite as physical or taxing? Instead of soccer, maybe you can play golf or participate in other low-impact or no-impact sports or activities, including: swimming, bicycling, walking, yoga, and fishing.

It may not be your first choice, but arthritis requires that you adjust and adapt. It is important that you stay involved in something. Stay active to the level that is appropriate for your physical condition.

Alert

Almost 44 percent of adults with doctor-diagnosed arthritis report no leisure-time physical activity. About 36 percent of adults without arthritis report no leisure-time physical activity, according to the CDC.

Doing All You Can Do to Stay in the Game

Have you done all you can do to stay in your sport of choice? Have you tried medication adjustments or local steroid injections to relieve pain and improve joint health? Physical therapy, hydrotherapy, wrapping, and splinting can also stabilize your joints and keep you in the game longer. Talk to your doctor and perhaps ask for a consultation with a sports-medicine specialist or orthopedic surgeon.

At some point, especially if your hips or knees are severely arthritic, joint replacement surgery may be advisable for you. The outcomes of joint replacement surgery, especially of the hips and knees, are highly successful and many patients achieve complete pain relief. A successful surgery may allow you to remain active in the sport of your choice.

The statistics show that having arthritis interferes with physical activity. To remain active:

- Consult with your doctor and take all steps to improve your health.
- Be realistic about what you can and cannot do.
- Look for alternative activities that will be fulfilling.
- Don't focus on what you have had to give up; focus on what you're doing now.

Turn a Negative into a Positive

It's sad to have to give something up. In the case of sports, you can find a way to continue enjoying sports. You can still participate, just in a different way. Make the sporting event a social event, for instance by hosting a party after the event. See if your enthusiasm for the sport can be channeled into fundraising, player recruitment, or coaching. Make a conscious effort to find a new role, one that is substantial and fulfilling for you. When you are forced to give something up that you are passionate about, you must find something of equal interest to fill the void. Ultimately, that's what new reality means— accepting the changes and making the best of your new situation.

Before you accept the changes, you may feel like grieving what you've lost. Don't be afraid to shed a tear, mope, or groan about it for a reasonable amount of time. At some point, though, time's up and you have to embrace your new reality.

CHAPTER 14

A Cyclone of Emotions

THE UNCERTAINTY THAT COMES WITH THE DIAGNOSIS of arthritis can be very unsettling. It's not unusual to fear what you don't know, and people who have been newly diagnosed with arthritis don't know what lies ahead. The possibility that life will change because of chronic pain and other symptoms of arthritis can lead to denial, anger, sadness, frustration, and other emotional responses. Positive attitude and positive actions can help you deal with your emotions, as well as the disease itself.

Fear—What Comes Next?

It's a question often asked, but with no definite answer. The course of arthritis varies from patient to patient. Following diagnostic tests and an initial evaluation by a rheumatologist, a course of treatment will be recommended. How well your arthritis will be controlled with the course of treatment cannot be predicted. Your doctor will schedule periodic appointments so your progress can be evaluated, and changes to your course of treatment will be made if necessary. It's all very scary and uncertain, especially at first.

You can take actions, outlined below, which will help temper the fear and anxiety that comes with not knowing the answer to these uncertainties:

- How you will cope
- How fast the disease will progress
- If you will become disabled

- If you can continue to work
- If you can care for yourself and your family
- What will change in day-to-day life

Alert

It's not uncommon for a newly diagnosed arthritis patient who has yet to learn about the disease to fear their mortality: The fear of dying crops up sooner rather than later. Learn about your disease and the adverse effects of treatments, as well as complications that can result. Become informed before jumping to conclusions about dying.

Finding Needed Support

Talk to your doctor openly about your fears. It may also help to find a support group for people with arthritis. Sharing your fears with people who are going through the same thing can be helpful because just feeling understood can relieve stress. If your fears are overwhelming and beyond the help which a support group can offer, don't hesitate to ask for a consultation with a psychologist. There are psychologists who specialize in helping people with chronic illnesses or other life-changing events.

Positive Actions

It's very hard to control fear and live with uncertainty. To cover up fear, some people unleash other emotions. Given that it's normal to be afraid and feel anxious about the future, it's unhealthy to be consumed by the fear. Give yourself the time it takes to adjust to your new diagnosis and grieve for your life before arthritis. It can't be done in a day, but you can set goals for yourself and work within your support system to accept the limitations which chronic arthritis imposes, realize you are doing all you can do with the guidance of medical professionals, never stop learning about the disease and treatment options, and focus on today by wrapping your mind around things you can do today.

The stress associated with fear can actually cause physical responses that will worsen your symptoms, including increased pain, muscle tension, fatigue, and more. Fear contributes to the stress-pain-stress cycle, which must be broken. It may seem like a job in itself, but each negative emotion should be replaced by a positive action such as patience, commitment, compliance, or perseverance. Build on the positive aspects. That is not to say negative feelings are not legitimate. For your better health, begin and end the day with hope—and that's not just self-help rhetoric—it's truly important.

Denial—This Is Not Happening

As a newly diagnosed arthritis patient, you may go into denial mode—it feels safe. After all, you don't have to deal with what you don't acknowledge. That may work loosely for some things, but not for being chronically ill. You do have to deal with it, so denial can only be a short-term coping mechanism, and can actually be detrimental if used as a long-term coping mechanism.

Long-Term Denial

Think about it: Denial over the long term is counterproductive. You should look for ways to cope with arthritis, not ways to avoid it. Arthritis is your new reality and having a positive attitude while being compliant with your treatment plan must be your goal. If you get stuck in denial, you won't be accepting your disease.

You must accept that you have arthritis if you are to focus on the things you should be doing to make you stronger and as healthy as possible. Denial is not only a distraction; if you deny the severity of your disease, you may ignore the small things that really make a difference in how you live and cope with arthritis.

Fact

> Denial is a defense mechanism in which a person is faced with a fact too painful to accept and chooses to reject it, insisting that it is not true despite overwhelming evidence. You may accept you have arthritis, but deny its seriousness.

Short-Term Denial

Short-term denial is not as harmful as long-term denial. It can act as a launching pad to get you where you need to be—facing reality and practicing positive actions. Short-term denial allows you that relatively brief period to adjust, almost like a car accident. If you are in a car that gets hit by another car, your first thoughts may be, "This can't be. This cannot be happening to me," but it doesn't take you long to get out of the car and deal with the situation. The quicker you start dealing with things, the faster you find some solutions.

How Can You Snap Out of Denial?

Support is huge in getting you out of denial. Recognizing denial is the first step; you have to first recognize you are in denial, then seek help or support. It can become more complicated if you deny the denial. Denying denial, simply put, means that you don't recognize you are in denial. If that's the case, you are three steps back from where you need to be in terms of coping mechanisms:

1. You are in denial.
2. You deny that you are in denial.
3. You think you don't need a doctor, a support group, or even need to acknowledge that you have arthritis and that it may change your life.

Accepting arthritis and facing the reality of the disease can be more easily achieved after you learn all you can possibly learn about the disease. Denial is rooted in fear, and it is knowledge that can ease your fear. You have to also believe that you don't need to hide from your new reality. Life with arthritis can still be a very good life.

Anger—Why Me?

Anger is a normal emotion that comes out of grieving for your prearthritis life. You loved your old life and now it's changing. How can you not be angry? There is nothing you knowingly did to cause arthritis, it just happened. So, along with anger, comes the "Why me?" syndrome. There are no concrete answers to these questions, at least none that would satisfy everyone. Some people of faith feel God has a plan for everyone, and without fully understanding it, they accept their lot in life. Others have a much more difficult time rationalizing "Why me?"

Anger can actually be channeled positively or negatively. If used positively, anger can be the catalyst for causing you to find solutions and better coping skills. Anger used negatively is resentful and can impede good coping skills.

How to Control Angry Feelings

If you don't learn to control or move beyond anger, it can make you irritable, stressed, and argumentative. You will need an outlet for the anger and it may range from minor outbursts to rage. Learning how to control your anger may include: meditation, guided imagery, exercise, yoga, and relaxation techniques.

Essential

Inspirational quotes are often helpful in redirecting your thinking. Consider keeping a journal of inspirational quotes you can read when you are feeling down.

Angry Ups and Downs

Arthritis is a variable disease, with ups and downs, flares and remissions. You can expect that if anger is one of your primary responses to arthritis, it too will have periods of ups and downs. That is why it's important to recognize that you're angry and learn to control the anger for your better health.

Coming to Terms with "Why Me?"

In your thinking, change "Why me" to "It is me." It won't help to dwell on things you cannot change. It helps to focus on your goals: Accept limitations, continue to learn about the disease, and focus on today. For some people, focusing on today doesn't even control anger—they're angry at today! In such cases, where anger has a veritable stranglehold on the patient, focusing on one or two specific positive people or events in their lives may provide a needed distraction.

Managing anger is important, even though a certain amount of anger is expected and normal. It can't be allowed to consume you and interfere with your life and well-being.

Why Are You Angry?

It's not hard to understand why some people get caught up in anger. Some people are angry: at the disease, at doctors for not having the cure, at the new reality, at the pain, and because of uncertainty.

It's a genuine emotion and it may be how you really feel. You only need to be sure it's not interfering with positive actions which will help control disease symptoms. Again, support groups or a consultation with a psychologist may help if your anger is beyond what you can manage yourself. There is no shame in needing a little help; arthritis is very difficult to live with successfully.

Sadness—You Liked Life the Way It Was

You can be rationally dissuaded from fear and denial, even anger possibly, but sadness is inherently part of living with disabling arthritis. Sadness should be accepted as part of living with chronic disease, but it should not consume you; sadness must be balanced with happy moments.

Bouts of sadness can be triggered by many things. Whatever makes you realize that life isn't the same and you can no longer do some things you once took for granted may provoke feelings of sadness.

Sadness can come from having difficulty with daily chores to having to rethink family traditions. The solution comes with downsizing. If it has become difficult to dust, vacuum, do laundry, and go grocery shopping all in one day, break your to-do list into manageable segments. If it's not possible to cook Thanksgiving dinner for fifteen guests, consider switching to a potluck Thanksgiving tradition, where each guest brings a dish.

Sadness will dissipate once you feel in control of your life again. Chronic illness makes you the priority: It's not selfish to view yourself as a priority, it's a necessity. Consider it self-preservation. Living your best possible life in spite of chronic illness requires that you take care of yourself, establish routines to keep your life structured, and create stability in your life so it feels less chaotic.

Is Sadness the Same as Depression?

Most people think of the physical changes and complications that come from living with a chronic illness, but the emotional effects are just as real. Sadness is rooted in loss, and for arthritis patients that means the loss of ability.

Essential

Tears are a physical response to sadness. Eighteenth-century French writer and philosopher Voltaire once said, "Tears are the silent language of grief." If you hold back tears, you are stifling your sadness.

Many people mistakenly think sadness and depression are the same. The reality is that sadness is a normal emotion that everyone experiences. Depression is persistent sadness that is often accompanied by feelings of hopelessness, helplessness, guilt, and even worthlessness. Sadness can be thought of as a mood, while depression is a medical condition. If you feel you have crossed over into true depression, get professional help.

Is Sadness a Permanent Condition?

Part of what causes sadness is the loss of independence and confidence. As you begin to need help with more and more things, your self-esteem can become eroded. The antidote for sadness is to impact your life in ways that will rebuild self-esteem and confidence. Once you give this serious thought and come up with a list of things you can do—things you feel will help you or help others—focus on those things.

Frustration—Losing Abilities

The loss of ability not only causes sadness, it can lead to frustration. It's as frustrating as it is sad when you can no longer do what you used to be able to do. You can't change the reality, but you can change your response to it.

If you focus on frustration, the unrelenting feelings will never subside, whereas if you focus on things you can do, feelings of frustration will become less strong.

Besides the things you can no longer do, it is frustrating to have to go to work in pain, have no energy, and feel constantly tired. You may be frustrated by the loss of normal range of motion in some joints and often feel sad, not wanting to socialize with family and friends. You may feel like your treatments aren't helping enough and you have no chance of getting better.

You're Not the Only One Who Is Frustrated

Arthritis affects you (the person who has been diagnosed with the disease) the most, but it also affects every person close to you. Your spouse feels the impact of your emotions intensely. In close relationships, if you are angry, your spouse can become angry too. If you are sad or frustrated, your spouse is likely to feel the same emotion. Similarly, it can affect your parents, your kids, and your best friends.

Realizing that you project your emotions onto those closest to you can make you feel responsible. However, you are not in this alone. Every person to whom you feel close wishes they could lessen your frustration. They take their cues from you, which is why it is so important for you to learn to overcome the frustration.

Remedies for Frustration

Instead of leaving the fix for frustration to chance, become more logical and practical. Ask yourself what you can do to help lessen the feelings of frustration. Make a list, if you think it will help, to keep track of useful ideas.

Don't let things remain undone. Using your household as an example, if there is a problem reaching things in your kitchen, a short-term fix is to have someone reach it for you. A more practical, long-term fix is to have pull-out shelves installed or lazy-Susan type shelves added to some cupboards.

If your yard is a mess and you can't rake leaves, the short-term fix is to have a family member or friend help you. Delegate the job to someone else. If you need a more permanent solution, consider hiring landscaping services or a responsible teenager from your neighborhood on a regular basis. The same scenario would apply to housecleaning and the need for a housekeeper.

There are myriad examples of how arthritis changes how you do things. You will begin to take pressure off of yourself and decrease your level of frustration when you train your mind not to focus on frustration, but rather on solutions. Instead of doing things yourself, shift to being a self-manager. As your own self-manager, you will focus on solution-based thinking.

If You Feel Different, You Are Different

So much changes with arthritis—are you even the same person? Chronic illness can shake your sense of self. If you let your self-esteem deflate, it is hard to revive it. You are not defined by what you can do, or by your abilities, or lack thereof. Your self-worth is derived from your personal characteristics, such as: sensitivity, compassion, perseverance, courage, and inner strength.

Alert

You need to know with certainty where you derive strength. For some people, it does come from within themselves. Other people turn to religion or spirituality. Finding that strength, no matter where it comes from, is what defines who you are.

Though arthritis may seem like the great destroyer at times, your inner self should remain intact. You are a mixture of those characteristics listed above. Arthritis, rather than destroying those, can make you reach within yourself more than ever before and depend on the power that comes from courage, perseverance, and inner strength.

It's complicated to think about and talk about, but if you look within yourself, you will find your inner strength. Simply put, arthritis may cause your physical being to become weaker, but it may also cause your inner self to become stronger.

To answer the original question—Are you a different person because of arthritis?—no, you aren't a different person, but your sense of self-reliance and inner strength may come from a different place now, impacted by different life experiences.

You will need strength to live with the chronic pain and physical challenges of arthritis. There may be very bad days when you want to crawl in bed and hope you never have to get back out. There may be days you feel like giving up. By tapping into your inner strength, you can change that feeling inside of you. Some people don't realize inner strength can be such a positive force in their lives. Relying on your own inner strength can have an almost magical effect by boosting self-esteem, confidence, courage, perseverance, and most importantly, your will.

Positive Thinking Matters

Maintaining positive thinking may be the absolute hardest aspect of living with arthritis. While you are dealing with the difficult issues related to arthritis, it's as big a challenge as any you face—to keep your mind wrapped around a positive attitude. How you think influences how you act. Accordingly, positive thinking leads to positive actions.

It's habitual, so getting on the right track with positive thinking is important. Positive thoughts get played over and over in your mind. Negative thoughts also can be played over and over in your mind, such as:

- It doesn't matter what I do—nothing's working.
- I see no results from the treatments I'm on.
- I want to be left alone.
- There's no point to my miserable life.
- I feel hopeless.

Essential

> Seek the help of medical professionals. Tell them if you are feeling pessimistic, hopeless, or unassertive. Together, develop goals and get excited about working toward a positive end. Feel victorious when you make positive changes.

Now comes the hard part: You have to consciously break the pattern of negative thinking by replacing each negative thought with a positive one. Take each of the above statements as an example. Change each statement to:

- It does matter what I do. I'll keep trying until something works.
- I must tell my doctor I'm not satisfied with the results of my treatments so he will help me figure out my next step.
- I need to be around people who I can talk to about how I feel.
- My life is good when I focus on things I can still do.
- I don't feel hopeless. I will never stop trying to get better.

Once you truly learn how to break the habit of negative thinking, you can control the cycle of negative thinking-stress-increased pain.

Goal Setting

Remember, you are a self-manager. You control how you think, what you feel, and what you should be doing. Start by setting goals: Consciously turn around any thought you recognize as contrary to what you have decided is good for your better health.

If you bear in mind that you control your thinking, and if you stop feeling like a victim of your disease, you will habitually become a positive thinker. Try an experiment: Spend a week or weekend grumbling, annoyed, pessimistic, and overwhelmed. Spend another week as the opposite. Which made you feel better overall? Getting positive thinking down pat is a big deal. Reward yourself for staying on track with positive thinking. Celebrate the victories—even small ones.

Finding the Courage You Need

You may hear at some point that another person thinks you are courageous for how you live and cope with arthritis. It does take courage to live day to day with chronic pain. Having courage means many things. It means you have:

- Faced your fears
- Focused on positive aspects of your life
- Prioritized your life
- Decided to work as long as you can
- Developed good communication
- Developed a positive rapport with your doctor
- Learned all about arthritis so you know what can happen in the future
- Decided unequivocally that you can handle living with arthritis

Even the most courageous can falter. To become a truly courageous person, you must know how to make adjustments quickly and get back to right thinking.

CHAPTER 15

You Need Understanding

GETTING UNDERSTANDING IS AS IMPORTANT as getting proper treatment for your disease. You need support and understanding from people closest to you because it's difficult to cope with the changes and adjustments required of living with chronic arthritis. If you are surrounded by people who don't understand what you are dealing with, it's an extra burden on you. Helping your family and peers understand helps you at the same time. Once they gain understanding, you will feel like you are all battling the disease together.

Helping Family Understand

It's most important for the people who live with you, your immediate family, to understand what you deal with on a daily basis. It sounds logical that your family should understand because of your daily interaction with them, but it's not that simple. Family members sometimes have the most difficulty understanding arthritis, and how it affects your life, because they may be in a state of denial all their own. Your family will grieve for how you were before developing arthritis, just as you do. In some ways, it can be even more difficult for them to understand because it's not their body going through it. Even so, the more your family understands about the disease and can offer you support, the more effectively all involved can deal with changes the disease imposes on your lives.

The Most Difficult Aspect of Arthritis to Understand

The most difficult aspect of arthritis for your family to understand is the variable nature of your symptoms. If you were to graph your pain or fatigue level on a daily basis, most patients would not produce a straight line. You may feel generally well for several days and without explanation your symptoms will flare. The variable disease course makes it hard to plan ahead, and requires that you and your family be flexible. Even when intellectually it all makes sense, it's hard to respond the right way without fail. Family members may struggle to reconcile certain aspects of chronic arthritis that become part of your life, such as:

- Severe fatigue
- Relentless pain
- Mood changes
- Depression
- Lack of spontaneity
- Disability

Family members may have difficulty distinguishing how your disease affects their role and your expectations of them. They need to adapt along with you. It's not uncommon for family members to feel like they don't know how to help you or what they can do for you. It's important for your family to realize that they are not spectators. Arthritis demands that the patient and every person with whom they interact closely be open to learning about the disease and how to adapt accordingly.

You Can Help Your Family Understand

Are you making the biggest mistake of all—expecting your family to understand without actively helping them to understand? It's so complicated for your family to know what to do for you and for you to know what to do for them. Family members often don't realize that you think they don't understand. The most effective tool for bridging the gap in understanding is communication. It's important for you and your family to express your sadness, frustration, anger, and other emotions. The worst thing that can happen is for either you or your family to feel you can't talk about it.

⌐, Essential

> The goal for any family living with arthritis is to live as normally as possible. Though life will certainly change, it is important to focus on positive aspects. Focus on things the family can do together. Find new activities to replace activities your family has had to give up.

Think of ways your family could gain understanding and make the suggestions. If you don't get an immediate response to your suggestions, don't give up. It may take more than one try to get your thinking across to them. Ask your family members to read articles, books, or Web sites which explain arthritis in understandable terms. Ask them to go to the doctor with you so they can ask questions or join you in attending support groups. Let them know that they can share their frustrations with you and communicate on a regular basis about how your disease is affecting them.

Beyond the practical ways you can help them understand, express to your family how much they help you by offering unconditional love and responding to your needs. It's different in each family. You may feel your family is not listening. You may feel they are overprotective. You may feel they are insensitive or that they don't help you enough. Whatever the issue or issues, it's imperative to talk about it, not just once, but as often as it takes until you feel you are all on the right track. Understanding arthritis is not an individual endeavor, it's a family endeavor.

Helping Friends Understand

You need understanding from your friends nearly as much as you do from your family. It's a bit different in that, typically, your friends don't live with you. It's actually a similar situation to that of extended family. The closeness and tight bond is shared, yet they don't see you on a daily basis like your immediate family. Friends may not be witness to your daily challenges.

The effect on friends is more social in nature. You may not be able to socialize or do as much with them as you once did. You may not feel like talking on the phone every day. You may be unable to go on shopping excursions at the pace you used to find invigorating. You may make plans and have to cancel at the last minute. "Party hearty" may be a phrase that no longer applies.

You Can Help Your Friends Understand

The answer lies in finding things you can still do together. The goal, as in all meaningful relationships, is to enjoy your time together irrespective of what you are doing. Even though you may have figured out what you need to do, you will have days when your friends don't understand. The advice given earlier in the chapter about helping family understand applies to your friends also. Ask your friends to follow the same steps listed above.

Draw from Your Friends' Compassionate Spirit

Your friends have fears, and feel sadness and frustration, too. It's common for your friends to feel anxious around you, not knowing how you will feel on any given day or at any given moment.

Alert

You may lose some friends because arthritis will affect your relationship. Not all people react or cope the same way. While this is a sad fact, realize it can also strengthen friendships. Arthritis, like many diseases, can sort out true friends from marginal friends.

Friends have different fears than you have. Your fears are practical: How will the disease change my life? When will I become disabled? Will I earn enough money? Friends wonder how your disease will impact your friendship. Realizing that you can't socialize as easily as you did before, your friends don't want to be shut out of your life. A true friend works at understanding and wants to help you and will also make all of the adaptations with you.

Helping Your Boss Understand

It's a unique relationship between you (the worker) and your boss. Your interaction is usually confined to your work. Once you are trained and can work independently, your boss depends on you to get the job done.

If arthritis is affecting your productivity, consider whether the difficulties you are having at work are apparent. In other words, do your boss and co-workers know why you have slowed down and why you aren't producing at your normal pace? Don't expect them to know what's wrong unless you have explained your health situation. Don't try to hide that you are having a problem at work. Concealment will just add to your stress level at work and exacerbate the problem. Besides, at some point, you probably aren't doing as well as you think at hiding it!

Does Your Boss Need a Crash Course in Arthritis?

Your boss won't understand your decreased production unless he understands arthritis. You can talk to your boss or give him some articles, books, or brochures to read, but typically he'll be more interested in finding solutions than in a crash course about arthritis.

Your work environment and work schedule are the two factors that may need adjustment because of arthritis. You will need support from your boss to get modifications made to either. You can request a better chair, desk, or any other equipment within reason that would help you continue work.

ADA Is On Your Side

According to the Americans with Disabilities Act of 1990 (ADA), your employer is required by law to provide reasonable accommodations.

Question

What is a "reasonable accommodation"?
Reasonable accommodation is "any change or adjustment to a job or work environment that permits a qualified applicant or employee with a disability to participate in the job application process, to perform the essential functions of a job, or to enjoy benefits and privileges of employment equal to those enjoyed by employees without disabilities." You can learn more about employment rights and the ADA at *www.eeoc.gov/facts/ada 18.html.*

Reasonable accommodation may include modifying equipment and work schedules, job restructuring, reassignment, and ensuring accessibility. With the realization that an employer, by law, is required to provide reasonable accommodation to an employee with a disability unless the employer can prove the accommodation would cause undue hardship, turn your boss into an advocate. Your goals are the same—you want to remain productive and your boss wants you to remain productive.

Keep your boss informed about how you are feeling and about any accommodations you feel would make a difference in your work ability. Good communication and a good rapport between you and your boss can make a huge difference at work. You need to feel like you can be open with your boss and your boss needs to feel you are still a dependable employee. As in any relationship, you need something from each other.

Helping Your Co-workers Understand

Working together is the key to a good co-worker relationship. Despite your illness and limitations, you can never leave your co-worker with the impression that you are lazy or that you are shirking your responsibilities. Without saying a word, your co-worker may notice your level of productivity has dropped, especially on certain days. Anticipate the questions before they're even asked, and be prepared to explain how arthritis is affecting your work.

Explain to your co-worker that having the job is as important to you as it is to them. Be open and honest while communicating with your co-worker. Draw upon your friendship and express how you need their support and understanding. Talk about the difficulty of juggling life at home and life at work. Gain their respect by telling them how you would deal with the situation if roles were reversed and your co-worker had arthritis and you were healthy.

Your co-worker may notice that you have given up breaks during the work day just to keep pace with everyone else or that you are using more sick days than usual. Your vacation time may go for recuperation rather than leisure activities. Co-workers will begin to notice and appreciate the sacrifices you are making just so you can keep working.

How Your Co-worker Can Help

Just as friends help one another, so it should be with co-workers. Small concessions can make a huge difference with regard to getting through the day. You may ask your co-worker to:

- Switch break times or lunch hours with you (for example, you may need to go earlier in the day)
- Keep the room temperature a little warmer for your comfort
- Let you have the more comfortable chair
- Trade a task (e.g., co-worker lifts heavy boxes and you answer the phone)
- Help you conserve energy by forming a car pool to work

There are so many ways a co-worker can help you if you develop an understanding. It's imperative for your co-worker to know you will never take advantage of their generosity and that you will return favors.

The Ideal Co-worker Relationship

You spend many hours a day at work. Some people spend more time at work than with their families. Like friends and family, co-workers also want to be able to help you and often don't know how. The ideal co-worker relationship should have a foundation of honesty, mutual respect, patience, understanding, and sharing. Your co-worker shares work space with you. By mere proximity, they are in it with you, but they are in it with you in a less literal way as well.

Don't be afraid of letting your supervisors know much you appreciate the kindness and consideration from your fellow co-workers—it's one way of paying back your co-workers. By telling your supervisors, you won't be diminishing your value at work, but instead, you will be enhancing everyone's value as a cohesive unit.

Fact

Flexibility is what will allow you to continue to work. In some cases, you may be able to do some of your work from home, especially if much of your work involves the telephone or computer. Consider all of your options.

Explaining Arthritis to Your Kids

Obviously, any tips or advice you are given about how to explain arthritis to your kids must be filtered through what you think is the best way to approach it. It's also dependent on the kids being old enough to learn about arthritis. Are your children old enough and mature enough to understand the human body?

If a parent has arthritis, kids are going to have questions even if they aren't old enough to articulate the questions. You, as a parent, are so in tune with your children you can likely read the expressions on their faces and know what they are thinking or what is troubling them.

Besides the age of the child (or adolescent), you should consider how afraid your child is with regard to what they observe. If your child was eight years old when you were diagnosed but they are ten years old now, your child is likely to notice some changes in you. Your child may wonder and wish they could ask:

- Why are you tired all of the time?
- Why don't you smile and laugh as much as you did before?
- Why are you in so much pain?
- Why do you walk funny?
- Why are you stiff after sitting through a movie?
- Why don't you walk the dog anymore?

Whatever your children considered normal, if it has changed, they have noticed, and may not know how to ask about it. Don't let that mislead you into thinking everything is fine with them. Just because they are not asking, doesn't mean they aren't worried and concerned.

It is often said that children absorb like a sponge. This is no different. All they know for sure is you, as their parent, are acting differently. It's difficult to allay their fears and explain in terms they would understand. Though it's difficult, you have to try to build understanding with your kids, even if it's not verbal understanding.

Start a Conversation

Try to engage your child in conversation so you can find out what they want to know about arthritis and encourage them to ask questions. Ask your children about arthritis to see how much they do or don't understand. Ask if they feel afraid because you have arthritis. It's important to confront their fears or other emotions. Ask if they want to go to the doctor with you and what activities they want to do with you for the next few weeks. (If they choose something you can no longer do, explain why you can no longer do it.). Decide together on a substitution for the activity you couldn't do. Let your child have input when choosing the alternate activity.

If your child is old enough to understand, encourage ongoing questions. You may have to explain something more than once. You must also "interview" them periodically so you can draw out of them what they know, what they feel, and what they are missing from you. It is vitally important to keep the conversation going. Even when you do that, don't expect your kids to fully understand at first. It will take time for them to grasp everything that's happening to their parent who is living with arthritis.

Comforting Children Not Able to Talk about It

I think you will agree that a conversation with a three-year-old about the pain of arthritis would be pretty much a one-sided conversation. You can't talk about arthritis until your child is at an age where they can comprehend concepts such as pain, fatigue, and sadness. You will need to explain in a way that doesn't scare your children.

Alert

It's important to comfort children. Do more of the things you still can do with your children and make it a priority to create great memories. Your young children will also learn from observing you. Your moods are reflected onto your children. They need to know everything is under control.

You may even choose to explain that arthritis is not only a disease of older people. It may help your children to meet with children who have arthritis so that they can relate to their peers. Contact your local chapter of the Arthritis Foundation to see if there is a support group for children with arthritis near you or if they can put you in contact with another family. Your children may begin to understand your arthritis better when they see it in someone their own age.

Dealing with Strangers and Acquaintances

It's different with strangers, neighbors, and acquaintances. They are not part of your daily existence, so your interaction is relatively minimal. You don't have enough time together to make a fleeting acquaintance understand arthritis, but you have to deal with them in a limited way.

Most people with arthritis choose to ignore strangers and acquaintances with whom they feel uneasy. That's certainly an option, but if ignoring leaves you unsatisfied, think of some "lines" you can use when the opportunity presents itself.

In a Restaurant

A lot of uneasy moments occur in restaurants. You may have staring eyes on you while trying to enjoy dinner in a restaurant. People may look at your hands if they are deformed or watch you get up from your chair awkwardly. It happens all too often. Most people feel it's best to ignore the staring. You don't know the person and you're unlikely to ever see them again. Others feel compelled to say something. If you are one who is inclined to speak, keep it brief and free of anger. Politely stop by their table and say, "I noticed you were staring at me. I have arthritis, but I'm doing very well. Thank you."

Essential

Remember, when you catch someone staring, you're not sure what is causing them to stare. Your first inclination may be to assume they are staring at your deformities or stiffness. They may actually be admiring how you handle it or may be remembering a loved one who suffered with arthritis.

In a Store

A store can seem like a racetrack at times. If arthritis has you moving in slow motion, you may feel you're in the way of people who are in a hurry. In this fast-paced world we live in, you have no chance of slowing down everyone else. The best options for you include going when it's less busy, letting people go ahead of you, using the disabled check-out lanes, and other commonsense solutions. Even planning ahead, you will encounter people who walk in front of you, bump your cart, huff and puff because you are too slow, and make you feel like you should have stayed home. You have to develop a thick skin when you have arthritis and not let such incidents bother you for longer than a split second.

Recognize, though, that there is a flip side to the negative encounters. You will meet even more people who are helpful and sensitive. You will have people offer to reach things for you, let you go first because they are not in a hurry, hold doors open for you, and generally be considerate. If you feel the need to say something, "I have arthritis. I appreciate your help" seems like an appropriate response.

Familiarity

There are other acquaintances you see on a regular basis. They aren't your friends or family, but they are not strangers either. For example, the receptionist at your doctor's office, your dental hygienist, your pharmacist, the waitress who serves you at your favorite eatery, your plumber, your hairstylist, and others who serve you and are familiar. You should develop a rapport with people who perform services for you. At some point, there is enough ease between you that letting them know you have arthritis may help them understand you even more. It may strengthen your bond and turn an acquaintance into a friend.

Dealing with Nurses and Caregivers

Your interaction with nurses at your doctor's office will become more familiar as you become a regular patient. The relationship becomes friendly and helpful. You depend on the nurses in much the same way you depend on your doctor.

📋 Fact

Study results have shown that if hospitals increased staffing of registered nurses and hours of nursing care per patient, more than 6,700 patient deaths and 4 million days of hospital care could be avoided each year, according to an article in the January/February 2006 *Health Affairs* journal.

In a hospital setting it's a bit different. Though nurses are professionals in any setting, the familiarity is lacking. Unless you have been hospitalized frequently and that's not likely, your nurse will not know the little things about you that can make a big difference. For example, if you have a painful right elbow with restricted range of motion, your nurse may extend that arm to put in an IV without realizing your other arm would be a better choice.

Nursing shortages have been a problem for years. In a hospital, the patient-to-nurse ratio is not optimal. Each nurse is taking care of more patients, and not that you aren't getting great care, but there is less time to become familiar. Once again, good communication is the answer.

When you are hospitalized, explain to your nurse which of your joints is most problematic. Explain why you can't move in a certain direction. Discuss why you make certain requests and have specific needs. If you are in the hospital following a hip replacement surgery, for example, you must have your call button in a place you can reach. You may not be able to move as quickly as other patients to get in or out of bed, to get on or off of a bedpan, to eat your meals, or to clean up in the morning. You may require more help than most patients. Be realistic with your expectations; however, don't expect your nurse to know what you need unless you have had a heart-to-heart talk. Don't expect that one nurse will relay your conversation to all of the other nurses—there's no time. Have the conversation with each nurse on each shift. Realize that you are not his only patient. Also, be respectful of how hard nurses work and their efforts to make you comfortable.

Don't expect your nurse to know everything there is to know about your specific type of arthritis. Nurses are not doctors; nurses carry out doctors' orders and specialize in caring for patients. Mutual respect and good communication will lead to understanding between you and your nurse.

The Financial Impact of Having Arthritis

ONE OF THE SEEMINGLY UNFAIR ASPECTS of living with chronic arthritis is that medical expenses increase and earning power may decrease. Some people with disabling forms of arthritis are forced to quit working and are left with applying for disability benefits. Not only does having enough money to live on become an issue, keeping health insurance is also an issue. Having finances in place to allow you to afford treatment and other forms of help you may need is important.

Will Your Earning Power Decline?

If arthritis forces you to reduce the hours you work or to change jobs, your earning level may go down. While it's hard to watch your earnings decrease, you have to focus on finding the help you need. You may feel like your options are spent, but there may be other options you have not yet considered.

If you feel concessions at work aren't enough to keep you at your current job and you haven't found any other job which you feel you can do, it may be the right time to apply for disability.

Here are some of the services that are available to help you if your current job will no longer work for your present situation:

- Government-sponsored vocational rehabilitation services
- Job Accommodation Network (JAN)
- Disability and Business Technical Assistance Centers (DBTACs)
- Small Business Self-Employment Service (SBSES)

Government-Sponsored Vocational Rehabilitation Services

The majority of people who have rheumatoid arthritis are eligible for vocational rehabilitation services that include counseling, testing, placement, resume preparation, interview skill enhancement, and financial assistance for education, training, and travel in connection with job placement. You can find more information on local government listings or Web sites. Also check for information at the U.S. Department of Labor (*www.dol.gov*).

Fact

Statistics show that more than one half of people who have rheumatoid arthritis become unable to work after ten years. Since 2.1 million people in the United States have rheumatoid arthritis, that means about 1 million people may face work disability.

Job Accommodation Network

The Job Accommodation Network is a free consulting service whose purpose is to increase the employability of people with disabilities. The service offers solutions regarding worksite accommodations, provides information regarding the ADA and other pertinent disability-related legislation, and provides information about self-employment options. For more information, you can call 800-526-7234 or visit their Web site (*www.jan.wvu.edu*).

Disability and Business Technical-Assistance Centers

There are ten regional centers, associated with the National Institute on Disability and Rehabilitation Research, which provide information, training, and technical assistance to people with disabilities, employers, and others with responsibilities under the ADA.

Each center works closely with local business, disability, government, rehabilitation, and other professional networks. More contact information can be found at their Web site (*www.adata.org/centers.aspx*).

Small Business Self-Employment Service

The Small Business Self-Employment Service, a service of the Office of Disability Employment Policy of the U.S. Department of Labor, offers information, counseling, and referrals about self-employment and the opportunity to start a small business. They can be contacted through the Job Accommodation Network at 800-526-7234 or at their Web site (*www.jan.wvu.edu/sbses*).

Check All of Your Options

There is likely much more help available than you knew about, and it's important to explore all avenues. In the United States, the Work Site (*www.ssa.gov/work/*) has information about the Ticket to Work Program, which helps people on Social Security disability go back to work and achieve their goals for employment. In the United Kingdom, similar help is available through WORKSTEP (*www.direct .gov.uk/en/DisabledPeople/Employmentsupport/WorkSchemesAnd Programmes/DG_4001973*). In Canada, WORKink is Canada's largest virtual employment resource center for job seekers with disabilities (*www.workink.com*).

Don't make decisions about quitting work before you are fully informed. Some people stay on the job longer than they should because they fear losing insurance benefits or fear never being able to work again. Money dilemmas can dictate and force decisions that are not necessarily the best for your health. On the contrary, some people quit work before they should because they feel unsure of various gradual step-down measures, such as reducing hours or taking a more sedentary position. They fear losing benefits because their value is diminishing as an employee and they fear being phased out by their employer. That's why it is so important to know your rights and your options.

Is Disability in Your Future?

The question is so important, yet the answer is so uncertain. It's one of the most common fears when you hear "You have arthritis." It's not only a worry because you are unsure if you will become disabled in the generic sense of the word, but also if you will meet the definition of disabled which would qualify you for Social Security disability benefits if you have to stop working.

There are definite requirements for Social Security disability. It's never too early to learn what the requirements are, just in case you ever find yourself close to needing the benefit.

Disability, as defined by the Social Security Administration, is "the inability to engage in any substantial gainful activity by reason of any medically determinable physical or mental impairment which can be expected to result in death or which has lasted or can be expected to last for a continuous period of less than twelve months."

To determine if you would qualify for Social Security disability benefits, answer these basic, preliminary questions:

- Are you currently working?
- Is your impairment or condition severe?
- Is your condition on the list of disabling impairments, per Social Security?
- Does your impairment affect your ability to do the work you have previously done?
- Can you do any other type of work?

Generally, if your earnings average more than the substantial gainful activity amount ($900 in 2007), as set by Social Security, you may not be considered disabled. Check all of the rules though, because some impairment-related work expenses (IRWE) can be counted.

Clearly, your impairments must interfere with basic work activities for you to be considered disabled by Social Security. If your condition is on their list of impairments, you will have an easier time qualifying. The lists are available online at *www.ssa.gov/disability/ professionals/bluebook/AdultListings.htm*. If your impairment or condition is not on the list, Social Security must decide if your impairment is of equal severity to an impairment that is listed.

Social Security also considers your ability to do the work you have done in the past fifteen years if your impairment is not on the list. If you can't do the previous work you were doing, Social Security considers your age, education, past work experience, or other skills that would enable you to do other work.

Question

What is residual functional capacity?
According to the Social Security Administration, "Your impairment or impairments, and any related symptoms, such as pain, may cause physical and mental limitations that affect what you can do in a work setting. Your residual functional capacity (RFC) is the most you can still do despite your limitations."

Residual functional capacity (RFC) is assessed by Social Security as part of the criteria used to determine disability. For applicants eighteen to forty-four years old, "less than sedentary" is the maximum allowed. For applicants forty-five to forty-nine years old, who are literate people of all education levels, "less than sedentary" is also the maximum allowed. The maximum RFC allowed for people over fifty years old increases to sedentary, light, or medium work.

If you believe you can no longer work, and if you and your doctors believe you would qualify for Social Security disability, you can begin the application process online (*www.ssa.gov/applyfordisability*). You can also request the Adult Disability Starter Kits online (*www.ssa.gov/disability/disability_starter_kits_adult_eng.htm*) or call Social Security with questions at 800-772-1213.

Even if you aren't ready for Social Security disability at this point, you will gain from learning about it. For example, besides the medical qualification, you have to earn enough work credits and have paid into Social Security to even be considered. You can find information about work-credit requirements online (*www.ssa.gov/ dibplan/dqualify2.htm*). If you worked long enough, find out how much you would earn if you were awarded disability benefits. You want no surprises—you must be informed. Did you know that once awarded Social Security benefits, there is a two-year wait before you are enrolled in Medicare? That fact brings up insurance concerns if you become disabled.

Insurance Concerns: Know Your Benefits

If you are considering a reduced work schedule or a different job, it's important for you to check on how that change would affect your existing benefits. Most jobs require full-time work status to be eligible for health insurance benefits and long-term or short-term disability benefits. If you were to change to part-time work status, it's possible that your benefits would be either lost or reduced. Once again, you want no surprises—be informed.

 Alert

It's hard to think about future disability while still wanting to work for as long as possible. Being realistic will help you down the road. If you have a disabling type of arthritis that may lead to living on disability payments, plan ahead for that inevitable day.

Knowing Your Benefits

To know how a change in work would affect your benefits, you need to know the details of what your benefits are now. Too many people don't take the time to investigate the details of their current benefits. Don't wait until you have to see a doctor or be hospitalized or need a prescription drug to know your share of the responsibility and what is paid by your health insurance plan. Learn about it before you need it. Also, don't wait to find out what would cause you to lose those benefits; learn about it before it becomes an issue.

Employers Can Change Health Plans

If you change jobs, your health plan may also change. Even as a long-term employee, your employer may change health plans, and it's important to find out how the change will impact you and your family. Is your doctor still on the list of providers with the new health plan? Have the deductibles and coverage changed? What provisions are there for a person like you who has a pre-existing condition? Try to avoid a lapse in coverage when changing insurance to decrease the likelihood of limiting coverage for pre-existing conditions.

Because you do have a chronic medical condition, all of these factors are much more critical to know than they are for the average healthy person.

HIPAA May Offer Protection

HIPAA, the Health Insurance Portability and Accountability Act of 1996, is a law designed in part to help you avoid the loss of benefits if you move from one group plan to another group plan. HIPAA states that group health plans cannot deny you based on your health status. HIPAA limits exclusion to health insurance based on pre-existing conditions if you change jobs or if you lose your job. In the event that you change or lose your job, HIPAA guarantees the availability and renewability of health coverage for some employees and individuals.

HIPAA also forbids the denial of coverage because of mental illness, genetic information, disability, or prior claims. HIPAA rules apply to all employer group health plans that have a minimum of two participants, and in some states, groups of one.

HIPAA's rules about insurance portability do not guarantee the same benefits, premiums, deductibles, or copays when moving from one group health plan to another. There are also rules that allow your current health coverage to be creditable within your new health plan: The time you were enrolled in the old plan is credited against an exclusionary period.

COBRA May Help

Many employees are unaware of COBRA benefits. According to the U.S. Department of Labor, COBRA, an acronym for Consolidated Omnibus Budget Reconciliation Act, ". . . provides certain former employees, retirees, spouses, former spouses, and dependent children the right to temporary continuation of health coverage at group rates. This coverage, however, is only available when coverage is lost due to certain specific events. Group health coverage for COBRA participants is usually more expensive than health coverage for active employees, since usually the employer pays a part of the premium for active employees while COBRA participants generally pay the entire premium themselves. It is ordinarily less expensive, though, than individual health coverage." You can find more important information about what qualifies a person for COBRA online (*www.dol.gov/ebsa/faqs/faq_consumer_cobra.html*).

Affording Prescription Drugs and Medical Care

The price of prescription drugs continues to go up, and finding ways to save on what can be a big expense, especially if you take several medications, is necessary. There are several ways you can save on prescription drugs, but you have to be conscientious about making choices that are not only cost-effective, but safe.

Generic Versus Brand-Name Drugs

There is considerable savings in using generic drugs. If you are open to using generic versions of your prescribed medications when available, make sure your doctor marks "Substitution Allowed" on your written prescription. You can also let your pharmacy know you want generic drugs when available. Actually, some pharmacies automatically fill prescriptions with generic equivalents unless specifically requested to use brand names instead. Check with your pharmacist to be sure you understand their policy regarding generic drugs. If you have prescription drug coverage, your copay will be less for generic drugs. If you pay out of pocket for all of your prescription drugs, the savings for generic versus brand-name drugs is significant.

Fact

The Agency for Healthcare Research and Quality (AHRQ) reports that between 1999 and 2003, the amount spent on brand-name drugs increased from $75.5 billion to $141 billion. The amount spent on generic drugs increased from $19 billion to $37 billion.

Price Breaks

It's not commonly known that larger quantities of pills are often given a price break. A ninety-day supply compared to a thirty-day supply can offer you considerable savings. Pharmacies also offer savings on drugs that are commonly stocked. Sometimes you can purchase the higher strength of a certain medication because it is cheaper and break it in half. This doesn't always work, however. In the case of enteric-coated medications, pill splitting can interfere with the way the medication works. Discuss this option with your doctor.

Choice of Pharmacy

As with anything, shopping around will save you money on prescriptions. It can be difficult to call around for price quotes from local pharmacies because they are so busy. Also, if you have prescription-drug coverage, the pharmacy must run it through your insurance to obtain a price. If you are going to shop around and compare prices, prepare a list of your medications and give it to the pharmacy so they can look up prices for you when they have time. The information is obtainable, you just need to allow time and be patient.

While shopping around, remember that sticking to one pharmacy has benefits. Keeping all of your medications at one pharmacy helps to minimize the chance of pharmacy errors and helps detect drug interactions. Consider all factors, including safety and convenience, when looking for less expensive prescription medications.

Government Programs for Prescription Drugs

If you qualify for Medicare, the Medicare Part D prescription drug plan is available to you. As a Medicare beneficiary, you may choose to enroll in Medicare Part D and select from plans administered by private insurance companies. The various plans have different premiums, deductibles, copays, and drug formularies. The plans are somewhat complicated, and it's best to analyze your options initially on the Medicare Web site (*www.medicare.gov*). There, you can compare plans and gather more information about Medicare Part D.

You may also be able to get help with prescription drugs if you qualify for Medicaid, a program available to low-income individuals and families who are deemed eligible according to federal and state laws. Medicaid is a state-administered health-insurance program. You can find more information specific to your state regarding qualifications and rules (*www.cms.hhs.gov/MedicaidEligibility/01_Overview.asp*).

Prescription-Drug Assistance Programs

Patient-assistance programs help qualified persons who cannot afford prescription drugs obtain medications for free or very low cost. Qualified persons have no drug coverage through private or public insurance programs and meet specific financial criteria. The Partnership for Prescription Alliance is a resource for finding nearly 500 public and private patient-assistance programs, including over 150 programs offered by pharmaceutical companies. To access more information about the various programs, call 888-477-2669 or visit their Web site (*www.pparx.org/Intro.php*).

Affording Medical Care

Research conducted by the National Data Bank for Rheumatic Diseases (*www.arthritis-research.org*) revealed that more than 40 percent of rheumatoid arthritis patients have difficulty affording medical care. Of those who reported difficulty affording medical care, about 37 percent did not buy prescription drugs and about 7 percent went without recommended surgery. The research showed that patients who reported having difficulty affording medical care had high rates of work disability, earned less money, and had less household income.

The Cost of Adaptive Equipment

Adaptive equipment, which helps compensate for lost range of motion and functional disability caused by arthritis, can be extremely helpful. Some patients do not realize how much help is available by way of adaptive equipment. Other patients do not think adaptive equipment is affordable and assume such equipment carries a hefty price tag.

An occupational therapist can help determine your needs. Medicare and Medicaid will pay for the assessment through a certified home-health agency or the outpatient rehabilitation department of a hospital. Some equipment is covered by Medicare and Medicaid, but not all. You must pay for equipment not covered by insurance. Suppliers and providers of adaptive equipment usually know what is and what isn't covered by insurance.

Besides items like reachers, raised toilet seats, shower benches, and other equipment that is useful in the kitchen, bathroom, or bedroom, you may need to adapt your car or make your home more accessible to preserve your independence. If you are purchasing a new car, check with the manufacturer to see if there are programs offered to help pay for any adaptations you require. Similarly, if you are considering a remodel to make your home more accessible, check to see if you qualify for any loans or grants to help pay for the necessary work. The message here is check before you commit— there may be financial help available.

Your purchases, if not covered by insurance, may be counted as medical expenses on your federal income tax if your doctor prescribes the equipment for you. Consult with a tax preparer if you have questions.

If swimming is prescribed as treatment for your arthritis, the cost of constructing a home swimming pool may be partly deductible as a medical expense. It must be proven to the Internal Revenue Service that the pool is for therapeutic purposes and not recreational purposes if questioned. Similar rules would apply to hot tubs.

The Cost of Household Help

Disability will cost more in terms of caring for your living space, too. The financial impact reaches all areas of life, no exceptions. When family members can offer help it's invaluable, but not every arthritis patient has family in close proximity. You may need to pay for the extra help you need and that can be hard when money is already tight. Finding affordable help at a reasonable price is the obvious goal. You may need a housekeeper, handyman, and landscaper.

Unfortunately, people with disabilities fear being taken advantage of and having to pay higher prices than most people. It's harder for people with disabilities to deal with hired help, and yet their need is even greater. Finding dependable help is very important.

Be sure to check if the person you are hiring is licensed and insured by the company you contracted with. If you are hiring occasional workers, consider talking to an insurance professional to make sure you have enough liability coverage in your homeowners policy. If you hire someone to work in your home on a regularly scheduled basis, you may need to purchase a workers' compensation policy. If the person you are hiring will be driving your car, it is advisable to notify your car-insurance company.

This is probably beginning to sound outrageously expensive and unaffordable. Your choices will depend on what you can afford. Just don't make the mistake of skipping over insurance issues that could have disastrous financial consequences. More information is available through the Insurance Information Institute (*www.iii .org/individuals/other/insurance/householdhelp*).

CHAPTER 17

Living in a Normal World

THE GOAL OF EVERY PERSON LIVING WITH ARTHRITIS or another disability is to live as normally as possible. To do that, you must learn how to do things more efficiently and more easily. You must learn how to better organize and plan. You must learn what works best for you and then do it over and over. It's difficult for people with arthritis to give up a hobby or passion because of physical limitations. Perhaps there is no need to give up on anything; perhaps there is just a need to learn a new way.

Traveling with Arthritis

If you had a passion for traveling before you developed arthritis, you won't want the disease to stop you. As with everything, you will need to find ways to simplify the process so you can continue traveling, if that is your desire. Whether traveling by car, train, airplane, or cruise ship, some of the helpful hints apply to all. Other tips are more specific to your mode of transportation.

General Travel Tips

Think of everything you will need for your trip. Plan ahead is the most important tip of all.

You will always need to prepare for how many days you will be gone and make sure you take medications in an organizer that will help you remember to take your pills and when to take them. This is especially important if you are crossing into different time zones.

Also remember to bring extra pills, in case you are delayed for any reason and some snacks so you can be assured you won't have to take pills on an empty stomach.

If you are not staying with family or friends, be sure you reserve a hotel well in advance and confirm that the room is accessible. People with severe arthritis would most likely be more comfortable in handicapped-accessible rooms. Don't hesitate to inquire about walking distances to and from elevators and dining facilities. Ask about anything that will put your mind at ease. Ask more than once, to be sure you are being given consistent answers.

 Alert

It's very convenient and efficient to prepare a checklist of essential items you will keep and refer to each time you travel. By having a prepared checklist, you won't have to recall what you need to take and risk forgetting something when you travel.

Whatever you need at home, you will need when traveling. Do you use bathroom aids, dressing aids, extra pillows? Pack light, but remember necessities that help you manage your arthritis. Consider taking any items which would help you if your symptoms began to flare, such as a heating pad or cane. It's also a good idea to use luggage with wheels, for easier transport.

Traveling by Car

Road trips can take an extra toll if you will be spending a lot of time in the car within the span of a day. Plan for the inevitabilities associated with car travel. Be sure you have your car serviced before you travel so you won't face additional problems from mechanical failure. Just in case, keep your cell phone within reach. Plan frequent rest stops to minimize stiffness. You won't regret taking the extra time to ensure your comfort.

Have extra pillows or a lumbar cushion available so you can adjust your body position as needed. If you have difficulty removing a gas cap, purchase a gas-cap wrench, which has a bigger, ergonomic handle designed to help arthritic hands. Be realistic about how long you can drive or ride in a car—overdoing it will ruin your trip.

Traveling by Plane

Some people with disabilities fear going to the airport because of long lines and travel restrictions that have been in place since 9/11. You shouldn't have to give up airplane travel, but you do have to be well-prepared. The Web site for the Transportation Security Administration (TSA) will help you keep up with the list of permitted and prohibited items (*www.tsa.gov/travelers/airtravel/prohibited/ permitted-prohibited-items.shtm*), as well as other dos and don'ts.

The TSA also has a section for travelers with disabilities and medical conditions (*www.tsa.gov/travelers/airtravel/specialneeds/index .shtm*). The information is updated according to changes made, and it's important for you to check before you travel by airplane. Current information is available regarding what disability-related equipment is allowed beyond the security checkpoint once it is screened. Policies regarding removing shoes and carry-on requirements are also updated as necessary.

Other suggestions for airplane travel which may make your trip more comfortable:

- Book nonstop flights when possible to avoid the extra hassle of connecting flights.
- Allow extra time. Rushing through an airport will wear you out and risk injury.
- Request an aisle seat when making your reservation to allow yourself extra leg room.
- If you will have difficulty walking through the airport, request an airport wheelchair or assistance ahead of time by calling your airline. With advance notice, a wheelchair will be waiting for you when you land at your destination.

Tips for Bus, Train, or Cruise-Ship Travel

As with any mode of travel, prepare in advance. As it applies, inquire in advance about the location of restrooms, bedrooms, stairs, elevators, or the accessibility of aisles. Ask if there is staff or personnel available to offer any special assistance you may require. Inquire how medical emergencies are handled. Here are some further tips:

- Try to schedule trips that require fewer stops or less need to get off and on the bus, train, or ship.
- Try taking shorter excursions at first to see how well you manage.
- Travel with someone else when possible.
- Schedule trips during less hectic or slower travel times—avoid the holiday crush.

Don't let arthritis put unnecessary fear into traveling. Planning ahead and being prepared should make you less reluctant when it comes to traveling. Try to anticipate any problems you may have and find solutions ahead of time. Don't deny that you may have special needs while traveling, because denial may get you into trouble.

Shopping Tips

Cost is important when shopping, but so is convenience for people living with arthritis. You will want to concentrate on conserving your energy while shopping so it doesn't become overwhelming. Focus on what is most problematic for you about the shopping experience and look for ways to simplify.

Home delivery or online shopping may be solutions, but if you're going to do hands-on shopping, consider the following advice:

- Shop at stores that have motorized carts available.
- Use stores you are most familiar with so you can avoid extra walking to find items.

- Stock up on bulky items so you don't have to juggle them each time you shop.
- Have a list prepared, so you can get what you need and get out before you've lost your energy.
- Shop when stores are less busy. Having to dodge people and other shopping carts will surely wear you out faster.
- Take advantage of store personnel who offer to load your car for you.
- Ask packers to put frozen food items together, so when you get home those are carried in first and the rest can wait until you've taken a break.

When shopping in retail stores or discount stores, be aware of where elevators and restrooms are as you enter the store. Don't wait until you are becoming too fatigued to search for them. You will be glad to know in advance.

When shopping for gifts for other people, don't weigh yourself down by carrying an oversized purse. Take things out of your purse that you don't really need to lighten the load. Consider shipping gifts directly to the recipient so you don't have to carry the package. Browsing through stores can be fun, but it helps to know ahead of time what gifts you are thinking of buying. Again, make a list even if you choose to deviate from it at some point.

Essential

Each individual should take what fits their shopping style and personality from the shopping advice. It needs to be about what works best for you, by finding ways to minimize stress. Some people think regifting is a solution. If regifting causes you more stress, then it's not the best solution for you.

Consider, if appropriate, giving one kind of gift for all of the people on your list. For example, get everyone books or get everyone

CDs. Narrow your range of gift giving to make it easier on yourself. Consider giving gift cards. The gift card idea makes it easier on you, and the gift cards are usually well-received because people can ultimately get what they want.

Cooking/Kitchen Work

Most arthritis patients get comfort from eating a good meal, yet have difficulty spending a lot of time in the kitchen preparing the meal. It's important to use cooking techniques which are simple and efficient. Plan meals you enjoy, but plan at least several days ahead. Plan to prepare extra so you can freeze meals and have them ready for those days you don't feel like cooking.

There are myriad cooking gadgets—utensils with built-up handles, lightweight cookware, Teflon pots and pans, and more—which you may find easier to handle. If that's not what you have now, consider it an investment for your better health. If you surround yourself with an accessible kitchen space and arthritis-friendly equipment and dishes, you will be inclined to cook more often and eat better. Here are some kitchen and cooking tips:

- Your stove should have controls on the front of your range so you don't have to reach the back panel to turn it on or off.
- You can buy one of the electric cookware products (e.g., electric fry pan, electric wok, electric grill) and sit while cooking.
- In the summer, outdoor grilling also allows you to sit down while keeping an eye on the barbecue.
- By attaching small casters to the bottom of a cutting board, you can change it into a transporting board, to help you move heavy pots along your counter top to the sink or wherever necessary.
- Boil potatoes before peeling them.
- To peel hard-boiled eggs, run the eggs under cold water after they're done cooking. The shells come off without a struggle.

- To drain cooked spaghetti easily, some people put a colander in the cooking pot then add spaghetti. Once the spaghetti is done cooking, you just need to lift out the colander. There are also pasta pots with strainer holes in the lid.
- Slow cookers or Crock-Pots are very arthritis friendly.
- Use an electric knife to cut meat, especially large roasts.
- Get your store or butcher to pack meat in portions you will use so you don't have to cut them and divide them again before freezing.

Fact

Sign up for a newsletter from a Web site geared toward making cooking easier. You will get tips and recipes delivered to your e-mail, and you won't get stuck in the rut of making the same old meal too many times in any given week. For example, check out Busy Cooks at About.com (http://busycooks.about.com/).

Once you realize arthritis requires that you do things differently and more simply, don't be afraid to learn how to best accomplish simple living. The examples given only tap the surface of what's available to you. There is so much written about meals in minutes, in large part because busy men and women who work outside the home need that kind of help. You, as a person with chronic arthritis, benefit from the flood of information about quick cooking because you need the same kind of help in the kitchen.

Arthritis-Friendly Hobbies and Activities

The physical and emotional changes caused by living with chronic arthritis may make it necessary for you to change how you do many things, and even require you to give up some. The ultimate blow would be giving up a hobby or activity that is your passion, which hopefully doesn't have to happen. By modifying and adapting the activity, you can probably still participate.

Keeping active with a hobby or activity you enjoy helps your mental outlook, and also helps your range of motion, though it does not replace regular exercise. You have to be careful about overusing joints and increasing pain. At times you are active with your hobby, you may need to adjust analgesic medications. That's something to discuss with your doctor.

Essential

The Arthritis Foundation has suggested that hobbies have a positive effect on people with arthritis by diverting their attention away from pain and other problems associated with the disease. Studies have shown that hobbies have health benefits, both physical and psychological.

You may have more leisure time if you stop working. You will need to fill your time with activities you find relaxing and pleasurable. Many people with arthritis enjoy reading, gardening, playing cards, embroidery, and sewing to name just a few activities. Generally, you will find that adaptive equipment which helps you hold objects will make a big difference in how your hands feel after working at your hobby.

For instance, gardening is made easier by using long-handled garden tools to compensate for reaching. Ergonomic handles on trowels, hand-held hoes, and planting scoops make gardening tasks easier. Raised flower beds also eliminate bending, which is normally required while gardening. Perennial plants rather than annuals require less work.

You will be able to read longer if you rest your book on a level surface. If you like to read in bed, place the book against a wedge pillow or a book holder. Playing cards can be made easier by using card holders or automatic card shufflers.

Embroidery is more easily managed if you use embroidery hoops attached to frames or that can be clamped to a table. Crochet hooks and knitting needles can be hard to maneuver. A nifty trick is to take the sponge off of hair rollers and slip them over knitting needles to improve your grip. Self-threading sewing needles or sewing machines which have automatic threading features are great for people who love to sew.

Most people with hand arthritis have difficulty gripping. Items with bulkier handles work best, but if you need a quick or temporary solution, try wrapping bubble wrap around something you need to get a handle on. Gripping shelf liner is great for wrapping around thinner handles (e.g., artist tools, sketching pencils) to make them thicker. The shelf liner works well underneath anything that slips away, which is its actual intended use.

Before giving up your favorite hobby, be creative and innovative when trying to find alternative ways that will allow you to continue enjoying it. Ergonomic equipment has become very popular, so it is not that hard to find. Some hobbies like dancing or boating may be harder to continue. It's important not to give up a hobby unless you absolutely have no other option. It is critical to replace any activity or hobby you have to give up with another. You may be replacing it with a more sedentary activity in some cases, but it's important to occupy your time with something else you enjoy doing. Give yourself a chance to develop new passions. Your pain, stress, and negative emotions will be less if you keep yourself truly interested in one or more activities.

Asking for Help

Change is never easy, and finding new ways of doing things can be a challenge. However, you may find the most difficult aspect of living with arthritis is asking for help. Some people have an easier time asking for help than others. You may feel it's a strike against your independence. You may feel you are imposing on someone or being a burden. The harsh reality is that you need help and you need to adjust your thinking to find that acceptable.

Fact

> It may seem counterintuitive, but you're actually helping others when you ask for their help. People feel good about themselves when they help someone—it boosts their self-esteem and feelings of self-worth. A good deed benefits both the one receiving the help and the one offering the help.

Asking for help is not a sign of weakness; it's part of the human condition. Every person needs some help from time to time.

Your family and friends often don't know what to do and actually feel helpless. If they can relieve some of your pain and make things less difficult, they want to do just that. They want nothing more than to be able to help.

Only ask for help when you absolutely need it. Do what you can do first before asking for help. If asking is somehow embarrassing to you, do it discretely. The kindest thing you can do for the person from whom you need help is to give advance notice. Try not to surprise them with a to-do list. Usually, people who are given enough time to plan for it and adjust their own schedules genuinely don't mind helping.

Try to package together the chores you need help with so your helper can get more done in one visit. Be reasonable though; the more time that passes before you ask for help, the longer your list grows. Try to address things in a reasonable amount of time so that you don't overload your helper with things to do.

Most people only need a thank you to feel good about helping you. An expression of sincere appreciation is the only form of repayment necessary. If you feel compelled to do more than just offer a sincere thank you, do something special and memorable for the person. Send flowers, bake a pie, take the person to the movies, or buy their dog some dog treats. Choose a gesture that shows how much you value their time and friendship.

CHAPTER 18

Coping with Arthritis

HOW WELL YOU LIVE WITH ARTHRITIS will depend on how well you cope with the changes that having a chronic disease will impose on your life. There will be physical changes and emotional changes, and on any given day you will be dealing with both at the same time. Your response to treatment will in part control your pain level and other arthritis symptoms, but your approach to living with arthritis will also have a big impact on how well you do.

Learning to Live with Pain

You wake up with pain. You go to bed with pain. Activity makes it flare. Rest doesn't always help much. Day after day after day—it can be grueling. Yet you have to live your best life possible in spite of it.

Some people have a harder time than others learning to cope with chronic pain. People who feel out of control because of chronic pain are the ones who don't do as well. It's important to be consistent with actions which help you feel in control. You will help yourself cope with chronic pain if you:

- Find a doctor who understands how pain affects your life.
- Allow your thoughts and emotions to move away from the pain—however you can accomplish it.
- Assess on a regular basis whether you are doing all you can do to control pain associated with arthritis.
- Replace bad habits that exacerbate pain (e.g., poor sleep habits) with good habits that promote pain relief.

- Accept that pain is a disruption in your life, but never stop searching or discovering ways to minimize the disruption.
- Chronic pain lasts a lifetime, so you must make decisions that will have long-lasting positive effects.

Chronic Pain Studies

The above advice may sound great in theory, but it must truly be applied. A study led by Lance M. McCracken from the University of Chicago, published in the journal *Pain* in 1998, reported that acceptance of pain was associated with "lower pain intensity, less pain-related anxiety and avoidance, less depression, less physical and psychosocial disability, more daily uptime, and better work status."

Another study, published in the same journal in 1999 (Arnstein et al.), concluded that "the lack of belief in one's own ability to manage pain, cope and function despite persistent pain, is a significant predictor of the extent to which individuals with chronic pain become disabled and/or depressed."

The studies reinforce that goals for learning to live with chronic pain should focus on: reducing pain, improving function, and building upon the belief that you can cope (self-efficacy).

Never Give Up

Chronic pain can be relentless, and you may begin to feel nothing you do matters. Never give up. Expect to have bouts of pain that seem untouchable. Remember that you are like a football player that has to take the field for every game. Arthritis is no game, but the analogy still fits. You have to keep taking the field. Keep in mind that certain factors exacerbate pain, while other factors help block or control pain. Focus on the factors that help control pain, such as medication, physical activity or exercise, relaxation techniques, and distraction (e.g., humor, hobbies). Avoid whatever exacerbates the pain-stress-depression cycle.

Find What Works for You

Though it's helpful to learn what helps other chronic pain and arthritis patients cope with pain, it's important to figure out what works for you. Never allow yourself to feel overwhelmed or to believe you are out of options. If whatever pain-relieving technique has worked in the past has become less effective, you may have to add more weapons to fight pain.

Feeling defeated will consume energy you need to fight pain. It's easier to say than to do, but you must replace feelings of discouragement with courage, hopelessness with hopefulness, pessimism with optimism, and passivity with assertiveness. John Quincy Adams once said, "Patience and perseverance have a magical effect before which difficulties disappear and obstacles vanish."

Learning to Live with Fatigue

Fatigue is a major problem for people with arthritis, especially inflammatory types of arthritis. Arthritis pain can exacerbate sleep problems, and the reverse is also true—poor sleep can exacerbate arthritis pain. Sleep problems shouldn't be dismissed, because there are actions you can take to improve sleep and reduce fatigue.

What Contributes to Fatigue?

Arthritis patients are often easily fatigued by daily living tasks that seem effortless for healthy people. A flare in disease activity can be expected to increase fatigue. Other factors that are known to increase fatigue include:

Overdoing or pushing beyond your limits with activity— Remember that pain is a signal to stop. If you overdo, your body will respond with more pain and greater fatigue.

Disrupted sleep or insomnia—Pain and discomfort associated with arthritis can interfere with normal sleep patterns. Insomnia is a problem falling asleep or staying asleep.

Medication side effects—Medications used to treat arthritis symptoms can have a side effect of increasing fatigue. A dosage adjustment may help.

Anemia of chronic disease—Low red-cell counts or low hemoglobin are commonly associated with inflammatory types of arthritis. Fatigue can be a consequence of anemia.

Mental drain—The physical aspects of arthritis can be mentally and emotionally draining. Fatigue can be exacerbated by depression, sadness, and feelings of hopelessness.

 Fact

Knowing what contributes to fatigue will help you focus on solutions. Fatigue is a recognized symptom of arthritis and related conditions, yet studies have shown it is often overlooked. The newer biologics drugs help to reduce fatigue, dramatically in some patients.

What Helps to Reduce Fatigue?

Recognizing what causes fatigue and what makes it worse will guide you toward actions that will help you control the problem. Conserving energy is the primary goal for controlling fatigue. You will have to make a conscious effort to conserve energy, and in this busy world we live in it doesn't always come easy. To conserve energy, pace yourself. Balance rest and periods of activity. Also, be flexible. If you are having a bad day, readjust and reschedule. It's important to plan ahead. If you know a particular day will be hectic, be sure the evening hours or next day will be stress free. Finally, don't underestimate the importance of convenience. Organize your environment and your schedule so that conserving energy is a priority.

Although the physical toll of having arthritis is the reason you feel fatigued much of the time or have trouble sleeping, advice that applies to healthy persons with sleep problems may benefit you as well.

According to the National Institutes of Health, you should choose a sleep schedule and stick to it. Don't exercise too close to your bedtime and avoid caffeine in the late afternoon or evening. Avoid alcohol before bedtime and avoid large meals or drinking a lot of fluids late at night. Avoid medications with known side effects of keeping you awake. Late-afternoon or late-day naps may interfere with falling asleep at night. Relax and wind down before bedtime; take a warm bath or shower if it helps. Clear your sleep environment of distractions.

Again, it's most important to identify what makes fatigue worse and what makes it better. You will find it requires a delicate balance. Listen to your body and pay attention to signals. Getting good sleep regularly helps break the pain-fatigue-stress-depression cycle.

Learning to Live with Uncertainty

Most people, healthy or not, live with uncertainty in their lives. You may get a good job, marry a fine person, and have children, but you are never certain of what the future holds. There is an element of uncertainty inherent to living.

People who have chronic illnesses have another layer of uncertainty to deal with. Most people with chronic illnesses, if given the opportunity, would preview their life five, ten, fifteen, and twenty years down the road. You can't—so that's akin to wishing for what you know you can't have. Rather than focusing on the future, you should be focusing on the present.

Focus on what you can do now, as well as decisions that will have positive effects now (e.g., lose weight, exercise, good sleep). The positive effects that result from focusing on the present will hopefully carry over to the future.

What You Would Like to Know for Sure

The questions you may want to ask have no definitive answers: How long before you will become disabled? How long before you will have to stop working? How long will you be able to care for yourself? How long before you need more help? Will you become more disabled than your neighbor? Will it ever get better? The questions are rooted in feelings of anxiety. Uncertainty breeds anxiety.

Set Goals

Set realistic goals for how you can help yourself now. It's somewhat unhealthy to be preoccupied with the uncertain future, because that takes your efforts away from thinking in the present.

 Alert

Set goals about your current treatment regimen. Are you satisfied with the response you are having to treatment? If not, how long are you willing to wait before you deem the treatment unsatisfactory? Be prepared to adjust your current treatment plan when necessary.

You should plan for long-term security. Make financial decisions that will bring you a sense of financial security at some point. If losing your job and becoming disabled are your worst-case scenarios, plan for the day and hope it never comes.

If you think you may need a caregiver at some point, plan for the day. It may give you peace to make plans and prepare for every possible contingency, but is it practical to do that?

With eyes wide open, prepare for your future security, but live in the moment. Always focus on improving your current situation. Richard P. Feynman once said, "I can live with doubt and uncertainty. I think it's much more interesting to live not knowing than to have answers which might be wrong." Carpe diem!

Learning to Manage Stress

The demands of everyday life are often stressful. A certain amount of stress is expected, but having a chronic disease such as arthritis can compound normal stress to a level that can be overwhelming at times. The normal stress response is sometimes referred to as the fight-or-flight response. It is the body's way of physically getting ready to fight back against a stressor, or run from it.

Physical Effects of Stress

The body releases epinephrine from the adrenal gland when it is undergoing a stressful event. The hypothalamus is stimulated to release hormones that increase production of cortisol, and other physical events are initiated by the nervous system. Stress provokes true physical effects, not only emotional effects. When you are stressed, you may experience:

- Muscle tension
- Exhaustion
- Anxiety or feelings of nervousness
- Indigestion or loss of appetite
- Dizziness or headache
- Trouble falling asleep

When you have to go to work, run a household, take care of yourself and your family, and have quality time with friends and family all while you are in pain and feeling run down, arthritis adds an extra dimension to what is already a hectic pace. For people living with arthritis, too much stress can increase pain, fatigue, and depression and make it more difficult to cope with the extra burdens that come with having a chronic disease. Pain leads to stress and stress leads to more pain. It is a cycle you must consciously work to break.

Essential

Not all arthritis patients respond the same to stress. Interestingly, one study revealed that a middle-aged female rheumatoid arthritis patient went into remission following two unexpected deaths in her family. Another study concluded that stressful life events or bad childhood experiences couldn't be linked to the development of rheumatoid arthritis.

ReduceStress

Stress management techniques should be part of your arthritis treatment regimen. First and foremost, you need to be cognizant of what causes you to feel stressed. A diary that tracks stressors and physical symptoms in response to the stressor may help you cope with or prevent those situations going forward.

It's an individual thing: What causes stress for one person may not be stressful for you. What relieves stress for one person may not be a stress reliever for you. After identifying your own stressors, follow this advice to help relieve stress:

Vent—Talk to someone and let it out. Keep stress from building up by releasing emotions associated with stress. If you have no one to talk to, write in a journal. Journaling is a great way to get your emotions out. Researchers have found health benefits associated with writing in a journal for just twenty minutes a week over a period of four weeks.

Focus on positive actions—Get rid of stinkin' thinkin'. Focus on positive thinking and put your energy into things that build your self-esteem and self-image. Avoid thinking that promotes feelings of depression such as "I can't do it" or "It's more than I can handle."

Take responsibility—If you feel overwhelmed by stress, recognize that you have the power to do something about it. Learn to say no if you feel you've undertaken more than you can truly handle. Learn to recognize when your mood is changing and take action before you feel too depressed. Consciously make the effort to relax.

Simplify and organize—Managing your time more effectively will help you feel less stressed. Don't wear yourself down by doing too much in a day. Spread out your activities and chores and don't forget to schedule rest periods. It's up to you to set manageable goals.

Avoid the sedentary trap—It's easy for you to justify a sedentary lifestyle. You hurt, right? You can't do as much, right? Can't do as much doesn't mean you can't do anything, though. Studies have shown that yoga, Tai Chi, and regular exercise can reduce perceived stress levels.

Be healthy—Eat well, sleep well, avoid alcohol, stay away from carbs and sweets, and take time to employ relaxation techniques. Decide what you find relaxing and do it. Clear your mind, engage in a hobby, or enjoy simple pleasures like walking your dog or reading.

Many people with arthritis will attest to the fact that arthritis itself is stressful, and additional stress makes arthritis symptoms much worse. Be aware of how you respond to stress and be sure to control negative responses to stress for your better health.

Learning to Manage Depression and Anxiety

It's not unusual for you to feel depressed or anxious at times because of changes brought about by having chronic arthritis. Sadness, fear, guilt, anger, and anxiety are normal to a degree.

Depression is a term that is sometimes inappropriately used to refer to sadness or the blues. Depression and sadness are not the same, and it's important to recognize the difference.

Fact

According to the CDC, arthritis is strongly associated with major depression, with an attributable risk of 18.1 percent, most likely through its role in causing functional limitations.

Depression Symptoms and Risk Factors

It's important to recognize a true depressive disorder, because there is help available. If you have experienced any of the following symptoms on a daily basis for several weeks, talk to your doctor.

- Lack of interest in things you used to enjoy
- Feelings of restlessness
- Feelings of guilt
- Feelings of hopelessness
- Cognitive problems
- Extreme tiredness

- Significant change in appetite, weight loss, or weight gain
- Trouble sleeping or sleeping too much
- Other physical symptoms such as headache, digestive problems, sexual dysfunction

Also be aware of depression risk factors, which may include previous depressive episodes, especially before age forty; recent stressful events in your life; a family history of depression; alcohol or drug abuse; medical conditions; and lack of a support network.

Coping with Depression

Though you recognize now that temporary feelings of depression and anxiety are normal with chronic pain and arthritis, don't dismiss persistent symptoms of depression and anxiety which need attention. If depressive symptoms are interfering in your daily life, long before the symptoms cross over into thoughts of death or suicide, get professional help. Counseling and medications that help with depression can be lifesavers.

Don't allow yourself to get into the trap of feeling hopeless. Tap into your inner strength and strong will and truly believe that life can still be happy, pleasurable, productive, and fulfilling despite arthritis.

If you don't feel that way now or have had periods where you didn't feel that way, you may be wondering how to maintain that mindset. First of all, know that it's not always easy, especially when pain and arthritis symptoms are particularly bothersome. It helps to concentrate on what you know deep in your gut such as: It's okay to be imperfect. In a world in which beautiful, high energy, highly accomplished people are celebrated, it's not hard to feel "lesser than." Never forget that the courage it takes to live with chronic pain on a daily basis is itself something to be celebrated.

You are doing the best you can do. In spite of chronic joint symptoms associated with arthritis, you continue to do everything to the best of your ability. Though arthritis steals away parts of your life as you knew it before, there is still a lot about your life that is worth hanging onto and worth your enthusiasm.

Focus on what you can do and what you can change. Don't focus on what you have lost. In your mind, set free those things you have lost. You can easily find yourself depressed if you keep calling up images of how things used to be. Let go of those images. Focus on today and how to make today better; it's not a hopeless situation.

Learning to Adjust and Adapt

The way you used to do a task may no longer be physically possible. Your physical limitations will continually present new challenges. Quite literally, you have two choices, and one of them isn't much of a choice: You can assess what is interfering or intruding on the way you used to do something and find a solution. The other option is to give up before trying to problem-solve.

You will need to continually reinvent yourself and how you think. Accept that the person you were before arthritis is gone. Try not to give that person a second thought. Put your effort into learning to be the best person you can be under the circumstance of living with a chronic illness. Face your new reality and consciously adjust and adapt to that new reality.

Making Necessary Adjustments

What might need adjusting? Adjust and adapt everything that is no longer working for you. Consider how arthritis has affected your living space. Consider how arthritis has impacted your time. Consider how the disease has affected your close relationships. Don't forget to consider yourself—how has your "normal" existence been affected?

Adjust and adapt your environment—Create handicapped-accessible space. Consider every room that is hard to get into. Consider every piece of furniture that's no longer functional for you. Make sure you create an atmosphere that is calming and comfortable for you.

Adjust your schedules—If you can't keep up with schedules, meetings, or other commitments, you may have to reconsider your obligations. If you have to give up something you used to enjoy doing, fill that time slot with something you can still do. Don't allow a void to be created.

Adjust time spent with family and friends—Find a new routine that allows you to have quality time with family and friends. You may have to change the day you do things together or what you do together, but be sure that whatever you take away is replaced by something doable and enjoyable.

All adjustments should be made so you're not left feeling something or someone is neglected because of you. Concentrate not on taking things away, but on doing things differently.

It's also very important to make mental adjustments, not just physical adjustments: You should adjust your expectations.

How to Remain Inspired

Where you find inspiration is personal and unique to you. Your source of inspiration may not be mine, and vice versa. Generally speaking, you may feel inspired by people who continue to do great things despite facing major obstacles, and others who cause you to be awestruck by their ability to consistently overcome problems.

🔲 Essential

People often inspire other people. What is sometimes hard to believe is that you may serve as someone else's inspiration. People observe your courage and achievements against all odds and you give them pause.

People Inspire People

People that inspire usually have a very positive attitude, despite living with some sort of challenge or challenges. They keep coming back, stronger than ever, after being knocked down by their physical illness or other difficult circumstance. They are the ones who rise above it all. You can look to these people as personal heroes and try to emulate their strength of character. Lance Armstrong comes to mind. After battling cancer, he went on to win the Tour de France as he had been doing before developing cancer. Christopher Reeve despite his spinal cord injury, worked tirelessly from his wheelchair, and sometimes from a hospital bed, to make a difference in the lives of those living with paralysis and other disabilities. Pierre-Auguste Renoir, the famous French impressionist painter, continued to paint and produce beautiful art. He made adjustments when necessary, but carried on with his work even after becoming severely crippled. There are myriad examples of men and women who persevered.

Words Inspire People

Sometimes the wisdom of someone's words can inspire. Books of quotations or Web sites about quotations (*www.quotegarden.com*) can really affect you in a positive way. You may want to collect meaningful quotations in a journal or notebook. In times when you are feeling down, read through your saved quotations. The words will reinspire you over and over again.

- "Pain is inevitable. Suffering is optional." ~M. Kathleen Casey
- "We have no right to ask when sorrow comes, "Why did this happen to me?" unless we ask the same question for every moment of happiness that comes our way." ~Author Unknown
- "We must embrace pain and burn it as fuel for our journey." ~Kenji Miyazawa
- "To have become a deeper man is the privilege of those who have suffered." ~Oscar Wilde

Those quotations are a sampling of words that may touch and inspire you. It's more significant for you to search for quotes which have deep meaning for you.

Faith

Personal faith is yet another inspiration for many people who are dealing with pain and physical ailments. This is not to promote one religion over another, but only to suggest that your own belief system can serve as your source of inspiration. Many people gain strength and feel inspired by turning to their faith and spirituality. Once again, it's personal how you choose to inwardly or outwardly express your faith and beliefs.

CHAPTER 19

An Eye on the Future

PEOPLE LIVING WITH ARTHRITIS have a vested interest in research and clinical trials. A discovery that would make a difference in your life would be ideal. As research findings are reported, be sure you comprehend the pertinent part of the reports and stay away from promises that can't be kept. In the past decade, there have been many new drugs and treatments marketed for arthritis, indicating that progress has been made with respect to managing disease symptoms.

Close to a Cure?

Researchers are probably not as close to a cure as you would like them to be. Significant progress is being made, and advances in research are leading to better understanding of what causes inflammation and how joint damage and joint deformity can be reduced or prevented. The mechanisms involved in joint destruction are very complex. Perhaps most telling is a quote from Gary S. Firestein, M.D., a prominent researcher from the University of California, San Diego. Dr. Firestein said in the December 2006 *Arthritis Foundation Research Update*, with regard to advancements in rheumatoid arthritis research, "We have made improvements in management, but there is still a long way to go."

Be Wary of the Word Cure

Patients are eager for a cure—that's a fact! While researchers are committed to finding the scientific evidence that will lead to an arthritis cure, peddlers of unproven remedies tout their products as actual cures. Then there is the media, anxious to be first with a breaking health story. Put it all together and patients are left with the task of sorting information from misinformation.

It's not just obviously hokey stories in the tabloids that you need to be wary of—the ones that have an alien on the cover and a headline about an arthritis cure in the bottom right corner. There are other examples of media hype from sources that would be considered legitimate. A search of your favorite bookstore will yield such titles as:

- *There Is a Cure for Arthritis* (1988) by Paavo Airola, ND
- *The Arthritis Cure: The Medical Miracle That Can Halt, Reverse, and May Even Cure Osteoarthritis* (1997, 2004) by Jason Theodosakis, M.D.
- *The Super Aspirin Cure for Arthritis: What You Need to Know about the Breakthrough Drugs That Stop Pain and Reverse Arthritis Symptoms Without Side Effects* (1999) by Harris H. McIlwain, M.D., and Debra Fulghum Bruce
- *The Arthritis Cure Cookbook* (2000) by Brenda Adderly
- *A Doctor's Home Cure for Arthritis* (2002) by Giraud W. Campbell
- *The 30-Day Arthritis Cure* (2005) by Len Sands

There are many more examples, and many of the books become bestsellers. There may be valuable information in these books and others, but some consider the titles misleading, since there's no cure for arthritis to date.

Promising Research Raises Hopes

Another somewhat recent example of the stir to announce the cure for arthritis came in 2000, when findings regarding B-cell depletion therapy for rheumatoid arthritis were announced at that year's meeting of the American College of Rheumatology. B-cell depletion therapy was being tested in small clinical trials at the time and involved using three drugs, prednisolone, rituximab, and cyclophosphamide. A media frenzy occurred, which reported that B-cell depletion was the cure for arthritis, but rather quickly the media backpedaled on calling it a cure. An editorial in the *British Medical Journal* accused journalists of being irresponsible.

Dr. Jonathan C. Edwards, primary researcher for B-cell depletion, responded to criticism by saying, "The word *cure*, in the form 'possible cure' has been on my Web site for two years. Our treatment was specifically designed to be a cure, in contrast to all treatments for arthritis other than high dose chemotherapy and stem cell rescue. Robert Matthews (from the *Sunday Telegraph*) used the word appropriately. Others may not have. We have not claimed a cure, merely that we had set out to cure and that results so far are as good as we had hoped on the first attempt and extremely useful in the short term."

Again, the public was left to separate hype from hope. Until there is a true cure for the disease, you will need to continue separating hype from hope.

Stem Cell Research

Stem cell research is a buzzword which gets a lot of attention, especially around the time of political elections. Some people think it's used as a ploy for politicians jockeying for position. Other people cling to the hope attached to stem cell research, as they imagine a cure for the disease they live with, or a cure that would assure that their future grandchildren will never experience the same pain they have lived with. You can see how easily stem cell research becomes an emotional issue. People approach stem cell research as a political issue, religious issue, or quality of life issue. Regardless of how you approach it, you should fully understand it.

Stem Cell Transplants—The Cure?

Stem cell transplants have been studied in the United States, Europe, and Australia as a potentially promising treatment for lupus, rheumatoid arthritis, juvenile rheumatoid arthritis, and scleroderma. While stem cell transplants are promising for some patients, the treatment is not for every patient.

During a stem cell transplant, bone marrow is removed from the arthritis patient or from a healthy donor. When the bone marrow is removed from the patient with arthritis, it is called an autologous stem cell transplant. Bone marrow cells are removed from the bone marrow that was extracted. Stem cells are left which can grow and develop. At this point, the patient undergoes high-dose chemotherapy or radiation to rid cells from the bone marrow still in the body. When that step is complete, the purified stem cells from the bone marrow extraction are injected back into the body, where the intention is that they will repopulate the bone marrow with healthy cells and ultimately lead the patient to remission.

 Alert

The stem cell transplantation procedure is not for everyone. It has risks, since it suppresses the immune system significantly. The procedure is reserved for patients who have failed all other standard therapies and those with life-threatening conditions.

Due to the risks involved, 5 to 15 percent of all stem cell transplants result in death. Rheumatologists and researchers agree that long-term followup needs to take place before stem cell transplantation is considered a cure for arthritis. Some transplant recipients had a recurrence of the disease, though it came back milder.

Why the Debate over Stem Cell Research?

In an autologous stem cell transplant, which was just described, the stem cells are your own. With stem cell research, the source of stem cell lines is what is disputed. Let's review the terminology:

- Stem cells are unique from other cells of the body.
- Stem cells are unspecialized cells capable of renewing and dividing themselves.

- Though stem cells are unspecialized, they can develop into specialized cells.
- Embryonic stem cells are derived from eggs fertilized only in vitro and donated for research through informed consent.
- Adult stem cells are undifferentiated in a specific tissue or organ. They can renew themselves, and can differentiate into specialized cells of the tissue or organ.
- Adult stem cells are said to be less versatile than embryonic stem cells. Embryonic stem cells can become all types of cells in the body. Adult stem cells are limited to their tissue or origin.

Research on embryonic stem cells could lead scientists to understand how undifferentiated stem cells become differentiated. Supporters of embryonic stem cell research hope it will lead to cures for many diseases, including lupus, rheumatoid arthritis, scleroderma, and many others. Learn more about stem cell research at the NIH Web site devoted to it (*http://stemcells.nih.gov/index.asp*).

Gene Therapy

Gene therapy has been another promising area of arthritis research, but some wonder if it has now taken a back seat to the biologic drugs. Gene therapy is quite exciting when you consider the possibilities, but is in its infancy in terms of practical application.

Genes, estimated to number in the tens of thousands, play a significant role in the making of proteins. It is possible to identify genes, isolate the genes from cells, and copy them. Put into the cells of living organisms, the genes function the way they were intended.

What was just described is like a four-stage process: identify, isolate, copy, transfer. A vector is needed to carry the genes into the target cells. Complicated for sure, but remember the goal is to be able to transfer genes to humans so the proteins from the genes will treat or cure diseases.

Pittsburgh Trials

A sixty-eight-year-old woman, who was already scheduled to have surgery for knuckle replacements, agreed in April 1996 to allow orthopedic surgeons to remove the synovial membrane of one of her thumb joints, which they transferred to a sterile growth media in the laboratory. The cells reproduced, and some were genetically modified to carry a gene that blocks inflammation. In July, the surgeon injected two of the woman's knuckle joints with genetically modified cells and two untreated cells. About a week later, the woman had the intended knuckle replacement surgery. Tissue and fluid was kept to see if having the genetically modified cells was beneficial.

As described, this was the first groundbreaking gene therapy trial for rheumatoid arthritis. Afterward, over a period of a few years, eight other women underwent a similar procedure. No adverse effects were found, and that was the goal of the study—to assess safety.

German Trials

Around the same time as the Pittsburgh trials, researchers in Germany used an approach similar to the Pittsburgh researchers, but inserted their genetically modified cells a month, rather than a week, before surgery. Two people participated in the German trial in 2000, and it was found again that no adverse effects occurred and the injected cells functioned properly.

Michigan Trial

In 1999, a third rheumatoid arthritis gene therapy trial took place at the University of Michigan Medical Center. In this trial, a gene taken from a virus was used. After injecting the gene into living tissue, the gene enters some cells, causing them to make TK, an enzyme. TK is normally not present in human cells. The study participant then took gancyclovir, a drug not harmful to human cells. However, in cells that produced TK, gancyclovir is converted into something toxic to TK-producing cells. The goal of this approach would be to control thickening of the synovium.

Essential

> On July 17, 1996, the first FDA-approved gene-therapy trial for a non-lethal disease (in this case, for rheumatoid arthritis) took place at the University of Pittsburgh Medical Center. It was a phase I trial for the purpose of assessing the safety of the procedure.

Drugs in Development

For a period of about five years, beginning in 1998, several new arthritis drugs were marketed, including a brand new class of drugs known as the biologics. The success of the biologics has led patients to wonder what's coming next. What drugs are in the pipeline? The question is especially pertinent, since the newest medications are geared toward being more effective while having potentially fewer adverse effects.

What's in the Pipeline?

Some drug makers are developing their own biologic drugs, while others are testing their own versions of COX-2 inhibitors.

Some of the drugs being developed for rheumatoid arthritis include the following; Most likely, not all will make it to market.

Prograf (Tacrolimus)—Tacrolimus, an immunosuppressant, is approved for kidney- or liver-transplant patients to prevent rejection. Researchers believe Tacrolimus could help rheumatoid arthritis by interfering with T cells that cause inflammation.

CP-690550—Pfizer claims this drug may be more effective than already marketed TNF blockers. It has the advantage of being a pill and not an injection or infusion. Phase II trials are underway. The drug was born of the effort to create a new transplant drug.

Golimumab (CNTO 148)—Golimumab is a fully human anti-TNF alpha IgG1 monoclonal antibody that targets the soluble and membrane-bound form of TNF-alpha. It is being developed by Centocor and Schering-Plough.

Pegsunercept—Pegsunercept is a therapy being developed by Amgen as a possible rheumatoid arthritis treatment.

LymphoStat-B (Belimumab)—Lymphostat-B is a monoclonal antibody which acts by binding to B Lymphocyte Stimulator (BLyS) to inhibit the stimulation of B-cell development. The drug is being developed by Human Genome Sciences for potential use in treating lupus and rheumatoid arthritis.

Denosumab—Denosumab is a monoclonal antibody being developed by Amgen for use with bone loss conditions including osteoporosis and rheumatoid arthritis. Clinical trials have revealed increased bone mineral density.

Actemra (Tocilizumab)—Actemra, being developed by Chugai and Roche, is a first-in-class humanized anti-IL-6 receptor monoclonal antibody which is said to slow down joint damage in patients with early rheumatoid arthritis.

IL-6 Blockers—Excessive amounts of IL-6 (interleukin-6) can damage the joints of people with rheumatoid arthritis. Other rheumatoid arthritis symptoms such as fever and high platelet counts may be due to IL-6. Researchers are working to find out if blocking IL-6 would decrease joint damage.

 Fact

Drugs in development are just that—being developed. Early on, some have numbers, while others are referred to by generic names. It takes years to develop a drug before it is submitted for approval, and later is marketed.

Participating in Clinical Trials

At some point, your doctor may ask you if you want to participate in a clinical trial. Unless you are well-informed on the subject of clinical trials, it may either seem like a scary proposition or the chance of a lifetime.

Alert

People who agree to participate in clinical trials do so for different reasons, but there are benefits and risks associated with clinical trials that must be understood. Don't enter into it lightly, but don't disregard the benefit which could come from your participation.

Ask your doctor what he feels about how the trial will benefit you as opposed to being treated with medication that is already being used for your condition. Be aware that physicians may get a generous reimbursement from the pharmaceutical companies sponsoring the trial, so determine to the best of your ability that it is in your best interest to participate.

Some people choose to participate in clinical trials because they have failed all other standard treatments, while others are motivated by a responsibility to help find better treatments or a possible cure. It's a way to personally contribute to the effort. Still others are motivated because some companies will compensate patients to participate in their studies.

Clinical trials are human studies designed to evaluate the efficacy and safety of a possible new treatment before it can be recommended by regulatory agencies for approval and marketing. There are four phases of clinical trials:

- Phase I involves few study participants, and it is decided how and how much of a medication or treatment should be given.

- Phase-II trials study the effect of the experimental treatment on a specific disease.
- Phase-III trials compare the experimental treatment to what is considered standard treatment for the specific disease or condition.
- Phase-IV clinical trials study the effectiveness of the experimental drug in combination with other effective drugs, and are often begun after the drug has already received FDA approval and is being used in the marketplace.

Clinical trials can also be used to study a new diagnostic technique, options to improve quality of life for people with a specific disease or condition, and even options that may prevent the disease.

Study Criteria

In reading about clinical trials, you have likely seen the terms *placebo, randomized,* and *double-blind.* A placebo is a pill or treatment that has no active ingredients, used as a control group for the purpose of comparison. Randomized refers to the random way study participants are assigned to receive either the experimental drug or placebo. Double-blind means that neither the study participants nor the researchers know who is in the control group or who was assigned to the experimental group. A double-blind, randomized, placebo-controlled study is the highest standard for clinical trials.

The Risks and the Benefits

Rules and regulations have been established to protect study participants from risk as much as possible, but not all risk is avoidable because there is an element of the unknown involved in medical research. Researchers are required to give prospective study participants complete information about the planned protocol for the clinical trial. Participants are required to sign an informed consent before entering the trial that shows they realize and understand there are known and unknown risks involved, such as: There may be side effects that range from mildly unpleasant to fatal reactions; the experimental treatment may not be beneficial or effective for the study participant; and the protocol may be more rigorous than you originally thought.

There are benefits, too. Besides a willingness to help medical research, a study participant gains access to the newest treatment possibility and to medical experts. The study participant becomes involved in their health care and may be able to continue with the drug even after the study ends if they had a good response.

The Informed Consent

The FDA requires that study participants be informed about several things. When participating in a study you must be informed of the purpose of the study; whether the trial is studying an experimental drug or medical device; the time required for the entire study; what happens during the study; what the risks and benefits are; and other procedures you may wish to consider besides the treatment being studied. You'll also be informed of where to get medical help if you are hurt during the trial, your contact person should any problems arise, and the fact that you can quit at any time.

Finding Out about Trials

Many people are interested in becoming a study participant, but don't know how to start the process. Get your questions ready and then surf the Net for clinical-trial Web sites. The best ones are: ClinicalTrials.gov (*www.clinicaltrials.gov*), an interactive online database managed by the National Library of Medicine, and CenterWatch (*www.centerwatch.com*), which list government-sponsored trials as well as industry trials.

The bottom line about being a clinical trial participant: Be sure you understand all aspects of the trial you are considering, and be sure you know all of your rights as a study participant.

Advocating for More Research

You may think research is very important, and you may wish you could help advocate for more arthritis research dollars. Do you know how or where to start?

You can start as part of grassroots advocacy, where you commit to positively influencing your own life and your community, and to influencing government officials to make right decisions.

First, you must believe that you can make a difference.

Do advocacy work through your Arthritis Foundation or Arthritis Society. You will have more clout as part of an advocacy campaign than as an individual. You may have to make telephone calls or write e-mails or letters. You may choose to visit your elected officials in person to plead for their help. You will organize, and your efforts will go toward creating awareness about arthritis.

Essential

Every year the Arthritis Foundation hosts the Advocacy Summit (*www.arthritis.org/advocacy/Advocacy_Summit/default.asp*), which gives advocates a chance to rally together on Capitol Hill. You can attend workshops and network with fellow advocates. The summit allows you to meet with members of Congress and speak with them and members of their staff about arthritis awareness issues.

The Arthritis Foundation has a section devoted to advocacy (*www .arthritis.org/advocacy/priorities/priorities_contact.asp*), which helps guide you to your elected officials, offers advocacy tips, and even offers a writing sample to simplify your tasks. Your voice is needed.

Many people with arthritis see the wisdom in advocacy, yet they feel their single voice doesn't matter. On the contrary, everyone's voice matters, and more voices speaking in unison about a certain arthritis campaign can definitely be heard.

CHAPTER 20

Arthritis Advice

AT THIS POINT, YOU SHOULD HAVE A BETTER IDEA of what arthritis is, the importance of an accurate diagnosis, your treatment options, the importance of good communication with your doctor, and what to expect from living with a chronic disease. You now know about protecting your joints, the importance of regular exercise, and compliance with your treatment plan. You even realize that there are mental and emotional aspects attached to arthritis, not only physical aspects. How is your mindset? Are you ready to live courageously with arthritis? Consider these last bits of advice.

Think of Your Needs (That's Not Selfish!)

At the end of each day, ask yourself if you have done all you could that day to make yourself comfortable and relaxed. Did you:

- Take your medications on time?
- Do range-of-motion exercises?
- Use adaptive equipment to protect your joints?
- Eat healthy foods?
- Reduce your stress level and do an activity you find relaxing?
- Get enough sleep the night before?

If you answered yes to most of the self-assessment questions, you're on the right track. If you answered no, you may need to refocus on your needs.

Alert

Many people have a hard time focusing on their own needs. Think about all of the parents who put the needs of their children before their own. Think of all the career-oriented people who put work first. When you live with chronic arthritis, your needs must be considered a priority.

It may feel selfish to be thinking of what you need. It's not selfish, though. You actually will do more for your family, your friends, and your co-workers if you take good care of yourself. If you take the time each day to address your needs, you will actually have more energy for other people and other activities in the long run.

Shed the Guilt

Some people truly have a hard time taking time out of their day to tap into their comfort regimen. Rather than taking time to watch the DVD or sit in the hot tub, you may be inclined to finish folding the laundry or read your child one more story. That extra push to finish the laundry or read longer to your child can be rooted in guilt. You think you are not as "good" as you were before you developed arthritis. You may subconsciously, or consciously, think that if you push to finish that laundry or read that one extra story to your child you will feel better, mentally and physically. That hardly ever works. By putting other things before your comfort regimen, you have deferred relaxation and gained little to nothing. One extra load of laundry will not rid you of the guilt you feel. Relaxation or meditation may have helped you relinquish those negative thoughts, however.

Saying No to Others, Yes to Yourself

It is a hectic world, and the demands of daily life are great. When you factor in your chronic illness, it can become overwhelming. Your comfort regimen will help you feel less overwhelmed.

Your time and attention is divided among family, friends, work, and church—you have obligations to each. Because of arthritis, you may have a more difficult time meeting those obligations on certain days. It may actually come down to saying no to others and yes to yourself on some days.

Prioritize Your Daily Schedule

It's a hard fact to accept, but you can no longer do it all; arthritis affects your ability to be as active as you once were. You may remember a time when you got up early, worked all day, did your chores at home, went to the gym to work out, caught up on your e-mail correspondence, watched TV late into the night or socialized, and got a few hours of sleep before repeating the routine the next day. When you have arthritis, it dictates how much you can do in a day, and it may not be what you used to do.

To-do lists are a great way of deciding what you should be doing and in what order, especially until it becomes routine to think this way. When creating your to-do list, don't forget to allow time each day for your comfort regimen.

First, decide which things must be completed today. If you can delay something until later in the week or later that month, put it as a lower priority on your to-do list. Consider the consequences of not completing a task or activity today. Be reasonable in your assessment. Things with greater consequences must be moved to the top of your list.

Then, break your list into "must do," "should do," and "could do" categories. Consider positive consequences as well as negative consequences. How will it help you to get a task or activity accomplished today? Assess the things that repeatedly fall to the bottom of your list. Can those things be eliminated, or should they remain as low priority? Whatever you eliminate will allow you more time for other things. Revisit your list at the end of the day and reprioritize it for the next day.

⌐ Essential

Prioritizing is a good strategy for effective living in general, but even more so if you have a chronic illness and have to choose which activities require your attention. Since you will no longer be able to do it all, prioritizing your daily schedule becomes even more important.

Be Reasonable with Your Expectations

Lists are a great way of helping you organize your time. If you are unreasonable in your expectations, though, the list may add more stress, which is the opposite of what you are trying to do. Remember how many hours are in a day when you compose your list. Keep track of how much actual time you have committed to other things. In other words, don't make a to-do list that is undoable.

Take your twenty-four-hour day and consider: how much time you spend working per day, how much time you need to keep up with chores at home, how much time you need for leisure activities, and how much time you need to sleep each night to feel well the next day.

Don't forget that disease management should always be your top priority. It's a necessity for you to try to manage pain and other arthritis symptoms so you can give more of yourself to other things. If you allow yourself to rob time from sleep to do other things, don't expect not to pay for that in other ways.

Give Up Some Control

If you can no longer do everything yourself, deductive logic tells you that you may have to delegate to others or even hire professional help. Lawn care, handymen, housekeepers, babysitters, and others who can provide services will help more than you can imagine. The money it will cost will be paid back in many ways. Remember the importance of self-preservation. You may be inclined to think you cannot afford it, when, in reality, you can't afford not to do it.

If you can't bear to skip your turn car-pooling the kids, think again. Put yourself in another parent's shoes: Would you expect them to participate in the car-pool plan, or would you be happy to help them by taking their turn if you knew how much it would help them? When you switch roles in your mind, the right thing to do becomes clearer.

Pace Yourself in All Activities

It's important to pace yourself in all that you do. It's more effective for a person with arthritis to balance rest and activity. You will be able to accomplish as much, if not more, by pacing your activities. Think about it: Do you get farther by cleaning the house in one hour or by cleaning the house in two hours? Either way, you have achieved your goal of cleaning the house. By taking more time, you preserve energy you can devote to something else. If you rush and do too much in too little time, you will increase your level of fatigue, stress, and pain, and that may negatively impact your ability to do things the next day.

 Fact

It's important for you to listen to your body's signals. When you start to become tired, take a break. If taking a break doesn't help, stop for the day and allow your body time to recuperate. Overdoing will increase pain and fatigue, as well as depression.

Getting Done Fast—Is That Always Best?

You may think that rushing to get through your daily chores is best. You may think you will rest after you're done with your list of chores. It's actually better for you to space out your activities by alternating more strenuous activities with less strenuous activities. You will find that you can get more done with the alternating method than by plowing through and wearing yourself out.

When you are experiencing more pain or worsening of other arthritis symptoms, take everything you do more slowly. On those days, you may require more breaks and less activity. Again, listen to your body and make those adjustments as needed. You can return to a normal pace once aggravated symptoms begin to diminish.

Reassess Your Pace

You may plan to accomplish your daily or weekly goals at a predetermined pace, but in reality, you may have overestimated your ability for that day or week. Even with the best-laid plans, you may need to adapt and adjust your schedule. When creating a to-do list or schedule, always allow flexibility. Account for the fact that things may not go exactly as planned. Allow yourself the opportunity to slow your pace when you need to and shift what you have scheduled to another time.

Consider also that some things may need to be taken off your list. Planning ahead and pacing yourself will definitely help you achieve most of your goals. Upon re-evaluation, you may decide you can't attend the PTA meeting after all, or you don't have the time to contribute something to the church bake sale. Consciously pacing yourself will help you not miss the things you have labeled as high priorities: Reserve your time and energy for your child's soccer game or school play.

Surround Yourself with a Support Network

You will need support from other people. Chronic pain and arthritis complicates daily living, and surrounding yourself with a support network is as important as any other thing you do to help manage your disease. Your support network will help you in many ways, but primarily they will help you find solutions and make adjustments that will make life easier.

Communicate with Other People Who Have Arthritis

You will find that you have a special camaraderie with other people who have arthritis and face similar challenges. Who can understand what you deal with on a daily basis better than someone who shares your concerns?

Local support groups are a great way to meet other people with arthritis who live in your community. Shared experiences promote mutual understanding. In a support-group setting, you can socialize and learn from others at the same time. You will meet people who will understand you, want to help you, and befriend you.

Question

How can you find a local support group?
The Arthritis Foundation is divided into local chapters, and many of the local chapters can give you information about local support groups. You can find your local chapter online at ✎*www .arthritis.org/communities/Chapters/ChapDirectory.asp.* You can also check the event calendar in your community newspaper.

You may not be able to find a local support group close to where you live, especially if you're in a rural area. The Internet has created a network of support groups you may choose to consider joining. Some people prefer the convenience of online communities to local support groups. Online communities offer chat rooms and message boards. The message boards are usually accessible twenty-four hours a day, every day.

There are numerous online arthritis support communities. Find one that suits your personality and has a tone you find helpful and comforting. The arthritis forum at About.com (*arthritis.about.com/ mpboards.htm*) and the Arthritis Foundation discussion boards (*www.arthritis.org/communitiesnew/Forum/msgboard.aspx*) are just two examples. An online search will yield several other possibilities.

Talk to People in Whom You Can Confide
The frustrations that accompany living with a chronic disease will begin to build up if you don't vent. Among your family and friends, reach out to the individuals who are good listeners and those you

feel comfortable confiding in. Talking to people and sharing your innermost feelings is an effective way of decompressing.

Don't isolate yourself or think that you have to deal with the challenges of chronic arthritis by yourself. Identify the people you feel you can depend on to lend you an ear and don't be shy about letting them know how important that is to you. At the same time, don't take advantage of their willingness to support you. Be considerate: Don't call them when you know they are going to bed; don't make every conversation only about you; and ask about their lives and offer the same level of caring in return.

Balance Your Life

As you are prioritizing your schedule, thinking of your needs, pacing yourself, and getting support, would you say you are living a balanced life? There are many ways to view balance.

Balance implies that you are spending the appropriate amount of time on any given thing. Is your work life balanced with your home life? If it is out of balance, you may be working overtime frequently and as a result aren't home enough with your family.

Some people mistakenly believe balance means that you have a lot of free time. On the contrary, your days can be very full, but you can still feel in control.

When you feel in control of your life despite chronic illness, and when you have accepted that arthritis is part of your new reality, you have reached a state of balance. With that sense of balance, you will continue to make good decisions. You will become very good at knowing when to take a break, get support, ask for help, or readjust your priorities.

Example of an Unbalanced Life

If balance begins to slip away, it's important to recognize the signs so you can adjust quickly and get back on the right track. Life may be becoming unbalanced if you find yourself saying or thinking:

- I'm spending too much time at work.
- I haven't seen my friends in a long time.
- I'm long overdue for a vacation.
- Every minute is scheduled and I have no time for myself.
- I feel stressed and tired much of the time.
- I don't have time to breathe.
- A lot of people depend on me.
- I have missed many special events with family and friends.
- I've lost control of my time.
- All I do is go to the doctor.

Bring Your Life Back into Balance

If you don't feel in control of your time, you won't feel in control of your life. Intellectually, you know how to live a balanced life. Chaos can disrupt your intended plans for keeping life balanced, though.

If and when it happens that you feel unbalanced and out of control, go back to basics. Revert to what you know works for you.

How you are feeling physically correlates with living a balanced life. If you are not living a balanced life, you will feel more pain, fatigue, and stress, and other physical measures will be out of line. Do what it takes to regain control of your life.

There's More to Life than Medical Problems

It can be easy to fall into the trap of becoming consumed by illness and the desire to get well. Having a chronic disease means you are living with it every day and every night. You wake up thinking about it and you go to bed thinking about it. You think about arthritis many times during the day, even when doing other tasks or activities. You talk about arthritis with your doctor, with your support group, and with your family and friends. It can consume your thoughts if you let it.

If you do let arthritis consume your thinking, that contributes to a life out of balance. There is more to life than medical problems. Make sure you give equal time to thinking about current events or such things as how to make someone happy or what you can do for a friend.

Alert

Give thought to other meaningful things. Shed the mental burden of arthritis by not thinking about it at all for short periods of time. Train your mind to focus on other important things, too. Strive for the balance—even in how you think.

New Reality Doesn't Mean Bad Reality

When you hear the diagnosis of arthritis for the first time, your head feels heavy and you feel like your world has just been turned upside down. At that point, much of the shock comes from not knowing the realities of the disease and from not knowing what to expect.

As your doctor speaks, you hear phrases like "chronic disease," "will require treatment for the rest of your life," "not every patient achieves a remission," and "can't predict the course of your disease."

That's just enough information that you won't fully understand, but enough to make you think it's going to be bad! As you learn more about arthritis, and as you live longer with arthritis, you will learn that you must view being diagnosed with arthritis as your new reality.

Dealing with a New Reality

Arthritis is your new circumstance and you have to learn to live your best life with arthritis. Arthritis is now part of you. To make your new reality an acceptable reality, start with positive actions. Each was covered already in the book, but they bear repeating:

- Learn all you can about arthritis—become well informed. It's your new reality.
- Agree on a treatment plan with your doctor and be compliant.

- Make healthy choices—eat well, sleep well, stop smoking, and maintain ideal weight.
- Address your needs every day, both physical and mental.
- Create a comfort regimen and do all you can every day to feel better.
- Prioritize, pace yourself, and live a balanced life.
- Embrace the new you. Life may actually get better in some ways.

Take Time to Adjust

Even when you become accepting of the fact that life with arthritis can still be good, there will be many adjustments to make. You'll have to do things differently and make future decisions with your special needs in mind. It will take some people longer than others to make the necessary adjustments and to learn to live well with arthritis.

L. Essential

Accept that you have the disease. Accept that there will be adjustments. Accept that there will be frustrations, disappointments, and emotional moments. Internalize what you do know for sure: You can do this—you can live well with arthritis.

Stop looking back for the person you once were. Look forward. The part of your life yet to be lived lies in front of you. Patience, perseverance, and courage will get you through the tough times.

Life continues after an arthritis diagnosis. Consider it your job to learn to live your best life with arthritis. Robert Frost once said, "In three words I can sum up everything I've learned about life: It goes on."

Appendix A

Glossary

Abduction:
Movement of a limb away from the midline of the body.

Acetabulum:
The cup portion of the hip socket that sits in the pelvis.

Acetaminophen:
A commonly used analgesic medication containing no aspirin.

Acupressure:
Eastern medicine practice of applying pressure to certain sites called meridians, as opposed to inserting needles.

Acupuncture:
Ancient Chinese practice of inserting needles into specific points of the body for the purpose of healing and relieving pain.

Acute:
A disease or condition characterized by sudden onset and limited to short duration.

Adduction:
Movement of a limb toward the midline of the body.

Adrenal gland:
Small gland located at the top of the kidney producing hormones that regulate many body functions.

Aerobic exercise:
Vigorous exercise promoting the circulation of oxygen through the blood.

Analgesic:
A medication with pain-relieving properties.

Antibody:
An immunoglobulin or immune protein produced by white blood cells. Antibody production is triggered by the presence of an antigen.

Antigen:
A substance the body perceives as foreign that stimulates production of antibodies.

Antinuclear antibodies:
Antibodies directed against structures inside the nucleus of cells. The presence of antinuclear antibodies serves as markers for some rheumatic diseases.

Arthritis:
Inflammation of a joint.

Arthrocentesis:
A sterile procedure using a needle to obtain joint fluid.

Arthrodesis:
Surgical fusion of a joint.

Arthroplasty:
A surgical procedure to replace a joint with an artificial joint.

Arthroscopy:
A surgical technique using a thin tube-like instrument inserted into a joint to view and repair damage.

Aspiration:
See Arthrocentesis.

Autoantibody:
Antibody against the body's own tissues.

Autoimmune disease:
A disease in which the immune system of the body turns on itself, targeting its own tissues, joints, and organs.

Bacteria:
Single-cell microorganisms causing infection.

B-cell:
White blood cells that produce antibodies (immunoglobulins).

Biofeedback:
A treatment approach that measures physiological responses and trains the patient to control the responses. Used to relieve stress and various painful conditions.

Biologic-response modifier:
A substance used to stimulate or restore the ability of the immune system to fight disease.

Biologic therapy:
Treatments employing biologic-response modifiers.

Bursa:
A fluid-filled sac between tendon and bone or tendon and skin.

Capsaicin:
Found in topical creams, a chemical derived from peppers that has painkilling properties.

Carpal tunnel:
A tunnel in the underside of the wrist formed by bone and the transverse ligament that houses the median nerve.

Cartilage:
Tissue covering the ends of the bones in a joint, acting as a cushion.

Chiropractor:
A practitioner of chiropractic.

Clinical-research trial:
Human trials designed to evaluate the efficacy and safety of medications and medical devices yet to be approved.

Combination therapy:
When two or more medications are used in combination to treat a disease, as opposed to a single medication.

Comorbid condition:
Medical conditions occurring together.

Complement:
A complex system of proteins found in blood plasma that combine with antibodies to destroy foreign matter.

Connective tissue:
A type of tissue that supports and connects body structures.

Corticosteroid:
Steroid hormone made by the cortex of the adrenal gland.

Costochondritis:
Inflammation of the cartilage of the chest wall, cartilage of the sternum, and possibly cartilage of a rib. Pain mimics cardiac chest pain.

COX-2 inhibitor:
A drug that blocks the actions of COX-2 enzymes.

C-Reactive Protein (CRP):
An indicator of the presence and intensity of inflammation, not associated with a specific condition.

Crepitus:
A clinical symptom characterized by a peculiar crackling, crinkly, or grating feeling or sound under the skin, lungs, or in the joints.

Cyclooxygenase-1 (COX-1):
An enzyme important in the production of prostaglandins. Functions include protecting the stomach and maintaining blood flow to kidneys.

Cyclooxygenase-2 (COX-2):
An enzyme that speeds up production of prostaglandins. Plays a role in swelling and pain associated with arthritis.

Cytokine:
A protein produced by white blood cells, acting as a chemical messenger between cells, either to stimulate or inhibit cellular activity.

Cytoplasm:
The substance of a cell outside of the nucleus.

Degenerative joint disease:
Synonymous with osteoarthritis.

DMARDs:
Disease-modifying antirheumatic drugs; used to slow progression of rheumatoid arthritis or other forms of inflammatory arthritis.

DNA:
Deoxyribonucleic acid; the basis for encoding genetic information.

Double-blinded study:
Neither the study participants nor the researchers know who in the test groups got the medication with the active ingredients.

Efficacy:
Effectiveness of a drug or treatment.

Effusion:
An abnormal accumulation of fluid.

Embryonic stem cells:
Stems cells derived from the inner mass of cells of a young embryo.

Enbrel:
The first anti-TNF alpha drug approved for the treatment of rheumatoid arthritis in 1998.

Endorphins:
Natural painkillers produced by the nervous system.

Enzyme:
A protein that catalyzes or speeds up chemical reactions in living organisms.

Erosion:
Holes in bone or cartilage from chronic inflammation.

Erythema:
Redness of skin due to inflammation or drug reactions.

Erythrocyte sedimentation rate (ESR):
A laboratory test using a special tube to test the rate of falling red blood cells over a period of time. A high ESR is an indicator of inflammation.

Fatigue:
Lack of energy, tired, physically drained.

FDA:
The United States Food and Drug Administration; the federal agency that regulates food, drugs, and medical devices.

Flexibility exercise:
Exercises to prevent stiffness, such as muscle stretches.

Folic acid:
B vitamin prescribed for people who also take methotrexate, since methotrexate depletes folic acid.

Gait:
The way you walk. Stride.

Gene:
A sequence of chromosomal DNA.

Gene therapy:
Treatment of disease by replacing, altering, or supplementing a gene that is abnormal and causing disease.

Glucosamine:
A component of cartilage.

Health assessment questionnaire (HAQ):
Clinical assessment of quality of life for people living with rheumatoid arthritis. Also assesses difficulty with everyday tasks.

Heberden's node:
Calcified spur of the DIP joint of the finger seen with osteoarthritis.

Herbal remedy:
Medications derived from plants.

Heredity:
Genetic transmission from parent to child.

Human leukocyte antigen (HLA):
The histocompatibility system can also serve as genetic markers for rheumatic diseases.

Humira:
The third anti-TNF alpha drug approved for the treatment of rheumatoid arthritis. A fully human monoclonal antibody.

Hyaluronan:
Substance used for viscosupplementation injections.

Hydrotherapy:
Synonymous with water therapy or water exercise. The warmth and buoyancy of the water helps people with arthritis exercise.

Hyperuricemia:
Abnormally elevated level of uric acid in the blood.

IM:
Intramuscular.

Immune:
Protected against infection or foreign substances by antibodies.

Immune response:
Activation of the immune system against foreign substances (i.e., antigens).

Immune system:
A complex system that detects anything foreign to the body, and the organs and cells protecting the body from foreign substances and infection.

Immunocompromised:
Immune system impaired by disease.

Immunoglobulins:
Proteins that are antibodies.

Immunosuppressive agent:
Medication that halts immune system activity.

Infection:
The invasion and multiplication of bacteria, viruses, and parasites in the body.

Inflammation:
Localized redness, swelling, pain, and warmth due to infection or injury.

Interleukin:
Proteins that communicate between white blood cells.

Intravenous:
Into a vein. Given through a vein.

Isometric exercise:
Exercises that tighten muscle without moving joints.

Isotonic exercise:
Exercises that strengthen muscle by moving joints.

Joint:
The area where the ends of two bones come together, facilitating movement.

Joint aspiration:
See Arthrocentesis.

Joint replacement surgery:
Also known as arthroplasty. Replacing a joint with an artificial one.

Leukocyte:
A white blood cell.

Ligament:
A band of connective tissue connecting two bones.

Lymphocytes:
A type of white blood cell, including T and B cells.

Lymphoma:
A tumor of lymphoid tissue.

Macrophage:
A type of white blood cell that ingests foreign substances.

Median:
In the middle. The median nerve runs through the middle of the wrist.

Methotrexate:
A DMARD used to treat rheumatoid arthritis and some other rheumatic diseases.

Mixed connective tissue disease (MCTD):
A combination of systemic lupus erythematosus, scleroderma, and polymyositis.

Monoclonal antibody:
Antibodies produced in a laboratory that bind to specific cells. Made from a single clone of cells.

Monotherapy:
Use of a single treatment or medication.

Morning stiffness:
Characteristic of having rheumatoid arthritis; patients wake very stiff in their joints and it can take more than an hour to be relieved.

MRI:
Magnetic resonance imaging.

Musculoskeletal:
Of the skeletal system, including muscles, bones, tendons, ligaments, and cartilage.

Myalgia:
Muscle pain.

Myositis:
Inflammation of muscle tissue.

Narcotic:
Drugs that block pain by blocking signals from the central nervous system to the brain.

National Institutes of Health (NIH):
An agency in the United States devoted to medical research. Consists of twenty-four individual institutes.

Nephritis:
Inflammation of the kidney.

Nerve:
A fiber bundle using electrical and chemical signals to transmit sensory and motor information throughout the body.

NIAMS:
The National Institute of Arthritis and Musculoskeletal and Skin Diseases; a part of the NIH.

Nodule:
A collection of tissue that can be felt and can exist at any level of skin.

NSAIDs:
Nonsteroidal anti-inflammatory drugs; used to treat inflammation.

Nucleus:
The structure of the cell containing the chromosomes.

Obese:
People who are more than 20 percent over their ideal weight.

Occupational therapist:
A trained and licensed therapist who teaches patients how to relearn skills required for daily living tasks.

Opiate:
A medication derived from the opium poppy acting as narcotic sedatives, suppressing the central nervous system.

Opioids:
Synthetic narcotics that resemble natural opiates.

Orthovisc:
A substance used for viscosupplementation injections.

Osteophytes:
Bone spurs.

Osteoporosis:
Bone-thinning disease resulting in abnormally low bone mass.

Osteotomy:
Cutting into or through a bone to remove a part.

Palindromic rheumatism:
A type of joint inflammation where the affected joint changes periodically from one part of the body to another and back again.

Paraffin wax:
Hands are dipped into warm, melted paraffin wax to relieve pain and stiffness.

Parathyroid gland:
The gland that regulates calcium metabolism.

Pauciarticular:
Affects four or fewer joints.

Peripheral neuropathy:
Abnormal functioning of the nerves outside the spinal cord.

Pheresis:
Procedure where blood is filtered, separated, and a portion is returned to the patient.

Photosensitivity:
A medication side effect of conditions like lupus. Sensitivity of the skin to light.

Placebo:
A sugar pill or pill with no active ingredients, used in clinical trials as a control for comparative purposes.

Placebo effect:
The person receiving an inactive ingredient reports a decrease in symptoms.

Plasma:
The liquid portion of blood, without the red and white blood cells.

Podagra:
Gout in the big toe.

Polyarthritis:
Arthritis in many joints.

Polyarticular:
Involvement of many joints.

Polymyalgia rheumatica:
A condition affecting muscles and joints, characterized by pain and stiffness on both sides of the body, involving shoulders, arms, neck, and buttocks.

Polymyositis:
An inflammatory disease of the muscle.

Pronation:
Rotation of the arm or leg inward.

Prosorba:
Antibodies are removed from blood of a rheumatoid arthritis patient using a special filtering machine.

Prostaglandin:
A hormone-like substance that modulates inflammation as well as having other functions.

Prosthesis:
An artificial replacement for a joint or other body part.

Purines:
Proteins found in most foods and in all human tissues.

Quality of life:
A patient's ability to lead and enjoy a normal life and normal activities.

Radiograph:
An x-ray.

Randomized:
Determined by chance, as in a clinical trial.

Range of motion:
The full normal movement potential for a joint.

Refractory:
Resistant to treatment.

Regimen:
A planned course of action.

Remicade:
The second anti-TNF alpha drug approved for the treatment of rheumatoid arthritis. Administered by infusion.

Remission:
A period when symptoms subside.

Repetitive-stress injury:
An injury that develops following overuse of a joint or muscle.

Research, controlled:
A clinical trial comparing a treated group of study participants to a control group.

Restless leg syndrome:
Uncomfortable sensations in the legs while sitting or lying still, resulting in a painful condition.

Revision:
A surgery required to revise a previous joint replacement because of failure of the prosthesis.

Rheumatic disease:
Conditions characterized by pain and stiffness of joints and muscles.

Rheumatism:
An older term referring to painful conditions of muscles, bones, joints, and tendons.

Rheumatoid arthritis:
An inflammatory type of arthritis that is also classified as an autoimmune disease. The pattern of joints affected is usually symmetric.

Rheumatoid factor:
An antibody measurable in the blood. It is detectable in 80 percent of rheumatoid arthritis patients and used to help diagnose the condition.

Rheumatoid nodule:
Lumps of skin, usually around pressure points, common to rheumatoid arthritis patients.

Rheumatologist:
A medical doctor specializing in the diagnosis and treatment of arthritis and other related conditions.

Rheumatologist, pediatric:
A rheumatologist who specializes in treating children with arthritic conditions.

Rheumatology:
A specialty of internal medicine focusing on rheumatic diseases and conditions.

Salicylates:
A subgroup of NSAIDs that does include aspirin.

Scleritis:
Inflammation of the sclera (the white outer coat of the eyeball).

Sclerodactyly:
Localized thickening of the skin of the fingers and toes.

Sclerosis:
Localized hardening of the skin.

Sedimentation rate:
See Erythrocyte sedimentation rate.

Seronegative rheumatoid arthritis:
Rheumatoid arthritis patients who are negative for rheumatoid factor. About 20 percent of people with rheumatoid arthritis are seronegative.

Side effect:
Undesirable consequences of treatment.

Soft-tissue rheumatism:
Rheumatic conditions affecting the soft tissues of the body (bursitis, tendonitis).

Spirochete:
A bacterial organism with a spiral shape.

Spondylitis:
Inflammation of one or more vertebrates.

Spontaneous remission:
A disappearance of symptoms, usually rare and early in the disease.

Stem cell:
A cell which has the ability to grow into any of the body's cell types, of which there are more than 200. Stem cells are unspecialized cells.

Steroid:
Potent drugs used to relieve swelling and inflammation, such as prednisone and cortisone.

Subcutaneous:
Under the skin, as in an injection given under the skin.

Supination:
Rotation of the arm or leg outward.

Supplement:
Dietary supplements include vitamins, minerals, herbals, botanicals, amino acids, and enzymes.

Symmetric arthritis:
Arthritis affecting same joints on both sides of the body.

Symptom:
Subjective evidence of a disease or medical condition.

Syndrome:
A combination of signs and symptoms that together present a disease state.

Synovectomy:
Surgical removal of the synovium (lining of the joint).

Synovial fluid:
The slippery fluid that lubricates the joints.

Synovial lining:
The lining of the joints responsible for producing joint fluid.

Synovitis:
Inflammation of the synovial lining of the joints.

Synvisc:
One of the hyaluronates used for viscosupplementation injections.

Systemic disease:
Throughout the body, meaning organs as well as joints.

T cell:
A type of white blood cell made in the bone marrow, which migrates to the thymus gland, where it matures and differentiates into other types of T cells and plays a role in the immune system.

Temporomandibular Joint Syndrome (TMJ):
Causes pain in the jaw and in front of the ear.

Tendon:
Connects muscle to bone.

Therapeutic:
Of or relating to treatment.

Therapy:
Treatment of disease.

THR:
Total hip replacement.

Tick bite:
Bite from a bloodsucking parasitic insect; method of transmission for Lyme disease.

Tissue:
A layer of cells that have certain functions.

TKR:
Total knee replacement.

Tophi:
The plural of *tophus*, indicative of more than one.

Tophus:
A nodule comprised of uric acid crystals.

Topical creams:
Applied to the surface of the skin.

Tumor necrosis factor-alpha (TNF-alpha):
An inflammatory cytokine.

Ulcer:
Erosion of skin or of the mucous membrane.

Ulnar deviation:
Hand deformity associated with rheumatoid arthritis. The fingers drift in the opposite direction of the thumb or away from the thumb.

Uric acid:
A substance resulting from protein metabolism.

Uveitis:
Inflammation of the inner eye.

Vasculitis:
A group of diseases that cause inflammation of the blood vessels.

Viscosupplementation:
Injection of gel-like substances into a joint to supplement the viscous properties of synovial fluid.

Yoga:
Through movements and deep breathing, yoga brings together mind, body, and spirit.

National Organizations

American College of Rheumatology
1800 Century Place, Suite 250
Atlanta, GA 30345-4300
Phone: 404-633-3777
www.rheumatology.org

American Pain Society
4700 W. Lake Ave.
Glenview, IL 60025
Phone: 847-375-4715
www.ampainsoc.org

Arthritis Foundation
P.O. Box 7669
Atlanta, GA 30357-0669
Toll-free: 800-283-7800
www.arthritis.org

Lupus Foundation of America
2000 L Street, N.W., Suite 710
Washington, DC 20036
Phone: 202-349-1155
Toll-free: 800-558-0121
www.lupus.org

National Fibromyalgia Association
2121 S. Towne Centre Place
Suite 300
Anaheim, CA 92806
Phone: 714-921-0150
www.fmaware.org

National Osteoporosis Foundation
1232 22nd Street N.W.
Washington, D.C. 20037-1202
Phone: 202-223-2226
Toll-free: 800-231-4222
www.nof.org

Raynaud's Association
94 Mercer Ave.
Hartsdale, NY 10530
Phone: 914-946-5808
Toll-free: 800-280-8055
www.raynauds.org

Scleroderma Foundation
300 Rosewood Drive, Suite 105
Danvers, MA 01923
Phone: 978-463-5843
Toll-free: 800-722-HOPE (4673)
www.scleroderma.org

Sjögren's Syndrome Foundation
6707 Democracy Blvd.
Suite 325
Bethesda, MD 20817
Phone: 301-530-4420
Toll-free: 800-475-6473
www.sjogrens.org

Spondylitis Association of America
P.O. Box 5872
Sherman Oaks, CA 91413
Phone: 818-981-1616
Toll-free: 800-777-8189
www.spondylitis.org

Index